Petit Mal Epilepsy

A Search for the Precursors
of Wave-Spike Activity

Petit Mal Epilepsy

A Search for the Precursors of Wave–Spike Activity

Michael Myslobodsky

Department of Psychology
Tel-Aviv University
Ramat-Aviv, Israel

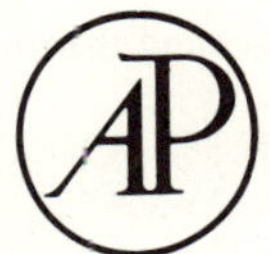

ACADEMIC PRESS New York San Francisco London 1976

A Subsidiary of Harcourt Brace Jovanovich, Publishers

ACADEMIC PRESS, INC.
111 Fifth Avenue, New York, New York 10003

United Kingdom Edition published by
ACADEMIC PRESS, INC. (LONDON) LTD.
24/28 Oval Road, London NW1

Library of Congress Cataloging in Publication Data

Myslobodsky, Michael
    Petit mal epilepsy.

    Bibliography: p.
    1.   Epilepsy.   2.   Diseases—Causes and theories of
causation.   3.   Diseases—Animal models.   I.   Title.
[DNLM: 1.   Epilepsy, petit mal.   WL385 M998p]
RC372.M95   616.8'53'071   75-36652
ISBN 0–12–511950–X

Contents

Preface

This book is intended for those interested in the use of conventional neurophysiological methods and theories for research in human brain pathology. It focuses on a unique rhythm—bisynchronous and generalized 3-per-second wave-and-spike activity—which is the EEG correlate of the petit mal fit. In effect, a study of this rhythm is a study of the nature of petit mal epilepsy itself.

The underlying assumption is that current neurophysiological techniques are not simply instruments for applied research: they also present theoretical problems that require extensive study. This approach necessitates occasional digression from applied neurophysiology into theoretical neurobiology to address such subjects as learning and reinforcement, asymmetry of the brain hemispheres, and the nature of evoked potentials. The border line between applied and basic research is sometimes very difficult to define, especially since experimental pathology is in itself an accepted method in neurobiological research.

The abnormal rhythm I intend to discuss in its theoretical aspect can be regarded as an instrument, or a way of producing the pathological hypertrophy of certain phenomena also observed in sound brains. The stability of these phenomena and the simplicity with which they are identified provide unique possibilities for experimental analysis of the bioelectrical activity of the human brain in general. This approach may be viewed as a study of normal brain activity via pathological reactions that lay bare the infrastructure of basic mechanisms governing the activity and interaction of the various nervous centers and their elements. A similar approach is the "monster method" in mathematics, in which the implications of a proposition are pursued ad absurdum in order to reveal the proposition's underlying error.

The approach is justified only when the disturbed normal function or process to be investigated is clearly defined, and this is essentially the only requirement of the method. It is easily fulfilled when the stages of derangement of the normal phenomenon being studied are determined. The same reasoning should apply to clinical studies. However, it appears that it is far more difficult to disclose by retrospective analysis the normal prototypes of phenomena distorted by disease. Small wonder, then, that the forms of rhythm basic to the development of the complexes of petit mal seizures have not as yet been determined.

In the clinical hierarchy of hypersynchronies, wave-and-spike episodes are the most benign. They are of short duration and have the least dramatic consequences to the life, health, and intellect of the individual. It would seem that pathological changes in the evolution of a rhythm should not make it impossible to recognize some features of the bioelectrical activity of the normal brain. Yet the rhythm of petit mal is so distinctive that it seems to be an entirely new phenomenon, unassociated with normal activity. Hence, the principal aims of the research detailed in this book are to discover normal precursors of wave-and-spike rhythms and to determine the conditions that facilitate hypersynchronization.

By the end of the nineteenth century, the previously existing corporative unanimity of physicians about the nature of what was called the *holy sickness* had ceased to exist. The writings at that time and later about the mechanisms of seizure contained a far greater number of hypotheses than was justified by the contemporary state of physiology, and notably, knowledge about the brain. As A. D. Speransky (1932) aptly said, "So much has been said about epilepsy that one would be justified in assuming that everything had been said about it." Yet the spate of books on epilepsy kept increasing.

Naturally, a clinical approach to research should limit possible interpretations of facts by testing the clinical viability of ideas developed in experimental studies. This primarily applies to generalized forms of epilepsy and particularly to short interruptions of consciousness (called *absences*)—for which no satisfactory models have as yet been created. Hence, I have also included a comparison of the mechanisms of the evolution of normal electric activity into the 3-per-second wave–spike pattern in the brains of animals with the mechanisms in the brains of humans.

The second task, determining what facilitates hypersynchronization, is a natural consequence of the first, which to all intents and purposes is simply a tribute to a half-forgotten tradition. Indeed, the idea that pathological discharges are but an intensification of normal ones was advanced at the dawn of electroencephalography. The idea of "increasing" alpha, beta, delta, and theta rhythms (Golla, Graham, & Walter, 1937; Penfield & Jasper, 1954) reflects this trend.

However, such dynamics were never properly proved, and the principle according to which "the disease intensifies, weakens or alters normal functions," advanced in Russian pathophysiology by A. D. Speransky (1932), is sometimes regarded as an anachronism. I was thrilled when I discovered that Niedermeyer (1966, 1972), a modern American researcher, is exploring this area.

This book proceeds from a study of experimental findings from research on animal models to an examination of the applicability of these findings to clinical research. It shows that the wave–spike discharge may emerge from the particular cerebral rhythm or the secondary evoked potential (Chapter 1). It demonstrates that conditions facilitating this metamorphosis may be created by lesioning the structures of the limbic–reticular system in mature animals (Chapter 1) or by irradiating them during a definite period of embryogeny (Chapter 2). It looks further for evidence of the similarity between experimental wave–spikes and their human prototype by exploring the properties of the former in behavioral experiments (Chapter 1), by investigating the treatment of animals with anticonvulsants (Chapter 2), and by analyzing animals' sensitivity to flickering light (Chapter 3). The relevance of these data to human pathology is investigated in a study of the reactivity of the human brain in normal subjects and in epileptic patients (Chapter 4). A general discussion of the problem is given in Chapter 5.

Obviously, in approaching an analysis of the 3-per-second bilaterally synchronous wave–spike pattern I am obliged to express my attitude toward the dominant centrencephalic theory of petit mal epilepsy. I do favor this theory, even though I propose a somewhat different version, which changes its essence. The ideas expressed in this book were published in Russian between 1964 and 1970 and are consonant with the theory developed by Gloor (1968–1972).

Acknowledgments

This book would never have been possible without the support of my friend Professor Irving Maltzman, of the University of California, Los Angeles. Without his encouragement and personal interest I might not have begun the ambitious undertaking of reviewing data published from 1964 to 1970. He also provided me with comfortable office space and his excellent library.

Gayle Boyd and Gloria Joyce have done a tremendous job of querying, proposing, and reorganizing the illustrations, as well as making unclear or clumsy writing comprehensible.

Professor Yu. Geinisman, now at Northwestern University Medical School, conducted neuromorphological studies described in this book. The contribution made by my collaborators and friends is reflected in references.

Finally, thanks are due to my students, who helped me prepare the manuscript. Matti Minz rendered invaluable assistance preparing graphs and putting the bibliography in order. Ina Weiner helped in assembling the references at a later stage. The illustrations were produced with the help of Jack Rattok. Leon Korb's efforts made it possible to finish this project more quickly.

1 Nature of Wave-Spike Discharges

SOME LIMITATIONS OF THE CENTRENCEPHALIC THEORY

I shall discuss here seizures belonging to the generalized category, but expressed almost exclusively by brief losses of consciousness (5–30 sec, rarely longer). These seizures have been named *minor seizures, petit mal,* or *absences.* Although all these names are generally accepted, I prefer the last, because the seizures are not usually attended by an expressed muscular reaction, an aura, or a postictal change of consciousness. Seizures of this type end as suddenly as they begin, and the individual is able to continue his conversation or work. Therefore, when speaking of minor seizures, I shall refer exclusively to this specific feature; other convulsive episodes, considered by some authors as part of petit mal, will not be discussed. I shall use the terms *petit mal, minor seizure,* and *absence* synonymously throughout this book.

From a clinician's viewpoint, there appear to be few grounds for the inclusion of absences in the group of epileptiform disturbances of consciousness, but there are a number of characteristics that support the classification. Chief among them is the unique imbalance of excitatory and inhibitory processes expressed in the special rhythm of the 3-per-second spike–wave (S–W) potentials that embrace the cortex during minor seizures. This rhythm may also signal an impending grand mal seizure.

Since 1947 there have been new developments in the study of minor seizures. These developments have come about through the predominance of a conceptual approach both pathophysiological and neurophysiological. This approach has been greatly advanced by an analysis of the electrographic correlate of the minor seizure—the 3-per-second S–W discharge, as described by Gibbs, Davis, and Lennox (1935).

The fact that these discharges are generalized and emerge synchronously suggests a connection with the activity of some structure in the central area of the brain having bilateral links with all neocortical fields (Jasper & Kershman, 1941). The nonspecific thalamus was regarded as the structure satisfying these requirements (Powell & Cowan, 1954). On the other hand, there are similarities in the disturbance of consciousness during epileptic seizures and that resulting from traumatic lesions of the rostral part of the brain stem. The optimal expression of the S–W complex occurs during slow-wave sleep—a fact that lends support to an argument for the existence of a center in the rostral brain stem critically essential for the preservation of consciousness.

Finally, it was discovered that bioelectric effects caused by stimulation of the nonspecific system have much in common with the S–W potential. The physiological studies of Moruzzi and Magoun (1949), Lindsley, Bowden, and Magoun (1949) point to the existence in the mesoencephalic–diencephalic region of a specialized system regulating both the state of consciousness and brain rhythm.

The fibers proceeding from the rostral thalamus are distributed predominantly to the orbitofrontal cortex and the structures of the limbic system (Nauta & Whitlock, 1954), which does not explain the emergence of S–W discharges in the areas of the neocortex not receiving direct projections from the intralaminar system. Even so, the facts and analogies noted became the basis for one of the most stable and fruitful conceptions—that of the centrencephalic origin of petit mal and, hence, of its electrographic correlate, the 3-per-second S–W discharge. From this point of view the cortical seizure activity is regarded as a passive response to discharges emerging in the rostral part of the brain stem (Penfield & Jasper, 1954). The presence of this phenomenon in the EEG became a weighty argument in favor of brain-stem pathology. At present the designations *centrencephalic* and *minor* are often used synonymously to describe absences.

It would seem that if further analysis of centrencephalic epilepsy is to be made, (1) the locus of the pacemaker of the abnormal rhythm should be clarified, and (2) action in that region should reproduce the electrographic and clinical picture of petit mal.

Jasper and Droogleever-Fortuyn (1947) began the search for structures whose stimulation would cause the cortical recruiting response. They succeeded in obtaining an evoked complex greatly resembling the petit mal potential by means of electric stimulation (with a frequency of 3Hz) of a small section of the intralaminar nuclei near the frontal part of the massa intermedia. It was later revealed that such stimulation in a cat results in the fixation of the eye and cessation of movement (Hunter & Jasper, 1949).

The period of intensive research launched by Jasper led to the disclosure of many important facts about the regulation of so-called "spike—wave" reactions of the thalamus. It was found that the spike is associated with the depolarization of most of the elements along the vertical of the cortex, whereas the wave is linked with the development of postsynaptic inhibition of the cell bodies. These discoveries were made "while pursuing a goal," but the goal itself was not obtained. All attempts to confirm that it is possible to induce a self-sustained wave—spike rhythm by stimulation of the oral pole of the brain stem proved unsuccessful.

As early as 1955 Ingvar (1955a), working with a preparation of the brain of an unanesthetized cat (or against the background of a weak Nembutal narcosis), emphasized that the termination of the stimulation of the centrencephalon may lead to the emergence of one or two slow waves. This was also observed by Jasper and Droogleever-Fortuyn (1947) following the termination of rhythmical stimulation. However, it would seem that we are dealing with a sort of ordinary off-effect that does not require any durable stimulation of specific frequency. Thus, the results obtained from the stimulation of the oral pole of the brain stem were no more than a banal rhythmic response of the cortex. Ingvar emphasized that the response could most easily be evoked by stimulation of the thalamus and the mesencephalic reticular formation. But in concluding a study in which about 4000 points of the centrencephalic system were stimulated, he wrote, "It has not been possible to establish the existence of a definable anatomical or functional—anatomical subcortical system consistent with any known such entity—which on electrical stimulation will produce a specific form of bilaterally symmetrical 3-per-second spike and wave potentials with a general cortical distribution [1955a, p. 150]."

This pessimistic conclusion led Ingvar to study isolated cortical islets, and he was able to induce S–W discharges with a frequency of 2.5–3.5 per second. Ingvar concluded that the cortex has at its disposal a net that is able to generate S–W discharges. However, he was not able to determine whether this circuit is activated without the participation of the subcortex and whether the discharges of the isolated cortex are identical with those of the intact cortex. I shall look into the matter somewhat later in this book. Pollen, Perot, and Reid (1963) and later Weir (1964) also thought it unlikely that the nonspecific nuclei of the thalamus participate in the organization of the S–W discharge. The stimulation of the intralaminar structures in a cat does not re-create the clinical symptoms of petit mal, and nonspecific thalamic nuclei are weakly developed in the human. Indeed, with the exception of the centrum medianum, they remain in a rudimentary state of development in humans, and in 30% of all cases the massa intermedia is absent (Crosby, Humphrey, & Lauer, 1962). Postmortem studies of these formations revealed no pathohistological changes on the level of the thalamus, basal ganglia, mesencephalon, or hippocampus (Cohn, 1968). Some patients suffering from genuine epilepsy did not have even rudimentary intra-laminar nuclei (Ajmone-Marsan, 1965).

In recent years there has been increased interest in the structures of the basal forebrain (including the orbitofrontal cortex) that are regarded as the rostral end of the powerful synchronizing system. Facts obtained mainly in the laboratories of Lindsley and Clemente throw new light on the classical views of the thalamic synchronizing system. The nonspecific thalamus is projected via the inferior thalamic peduncle (Scheibel & Scheibel, 1967) to the orbital cortex (Nauta & Whitlock, 1954) and forms an integral whole with it. In the cat, the bilateral removal of the orbital cortex eliminates the recruiting reaction and barbiturate spindle in the cortex as well as in the thalamus. Controlled destruction of areas adjacent to the orbital cortex did not evoke a similar effect (Velasco & Lindsley, 1965; Velasco, Skinner, Asaro, & Lindsley, 1968).

If the removal of the orbital cortex suppresses the recruiting spike, the prototype of the spike of the S–W complex in Jasper's model, then according to a simple syllogism destruction of the orbitofrontal cortex must also supress the S–W discharges evoked by irritation of the thalamus and, possibly, also the S–W discharges of other origin. This proposition was put forward by Villablanca, Schlag, and Marcus (1970). They evoked complexes of the S–W type by the intravenous injection of 12–25 mg/kg of chlorambucil and by the classical method of stimulation of the nucleus centrum medianum or nucleus reuniens with 3-Hz electrical pulses. They observed that the unilateral destruction of the inferior thalamic peduncle (the second hemisphere served as control) eliminated spindles in the homolateral hemisphere and markedly suppressed S–W complexes of thalamic origin (as also in the experiments carried out by Skinner & Lindsley, 1967).

This, however, is hardly unexpected. A suppression of S–W discharges resulting from the introduction of chlorambucil would have been surprising. However, these discharges were far less affected after the destruction of the inferior thalamic peduncle. Villablanca *et al.* associated the greater resistance of the pharmacologically evoked S–W complex with the action of chlorambucil on the cortex. They demonstrated this association in a special experiment on the isolated frontal cortex. Thus, the attempt to demonstrate the affinity of the S–W complex evoked by thalamic stimulation with discharges of other origin was essentially unsuccessful. In their discussion of the origin of the S–W discharges Villablanca *et al.* adopted a polycentric conception of centrencephalic epilepsy, although they did not brush aside the role of a potential thalamic pacemaker.

The destruction of a suspected pacemaker structure may not be the only cause for the suppression of S–W discharges and the complete elimination of spindles and the recruiting reaction following the removal of the orbitofrontal cortex. Powerful inhibitory pathways descend from the structures of the orbitofrontal cortex to the reticular formation of the brain stem, at least in cats (Clemente, 1968). Destroying the orbitofrontal cortex leads to the reciprocal release of the reticular activating system, which is accompanied by behavioral and EEG activation. It may be that the suppression of all forms of synchronized activity is based on this classical effect. In any case it is responsible for the disruption of those patterns extremely sensitive to the level of activation, such as the sigma rhythm, the recruiting response, and, to a certain degree, the S–W discharges.

Schlag (1967), commenting on the report of Skinner and Lindsley (1967) brushed aside this assumption when he quoted the results of control experiments he made with Villablanca. In these experiments involving four cats a full precollicular transection was made in addition to bilateral destruction of the inferior thalamic peduncle area. The EEG of this preparation registered neither spindle nor high-frequency activity; it displayed only irregular delta activity. Thus, it would seem that the suppression of the sigma rhythm is not connected with the release of the reticular activating system.

Robertson and Lynch (1971), who repeated these experiments, reached the opposite conclusion, that spindles do not disappear following the destruction of the orbitofrontal cortex if the reticular formation of the brain stem is damaged at the same time. In cats having an intact reticular formation the sigma rhythm disappeared after the removal of the orbitofrontal cortex but was regenerated as soon as small doses of Nembutal or scopolamine were introduced, or when the cat became quiet and drowsy.

Staunton and Sasaki (1971) were also unable to eliminate the sigma rhythm and the recruiting reaction by suction or cauterization of the orbitofrontal cortex. In these experiments Nembutal was also used, and recording of the spontaneous EEG and the recruiting response was intentionally made from cortical areas sufficiently distant from the injured tissue.

Feeney and Gullotta (1972) reported that in a cat anesthetized with Nembutal it was possible to abolish cortical spindles on the side of the rostral thalamic lesion. On the lesioned side they observed a reduction in the amplitude of both tonic and clonic Metrazol-induced grand mal seizure discharges. Although the same result was obtained in control unanesthetized preparations, it is less convincing because Feeney and Gullotta used a long-lasting local anesthetic (Xylocaine). Local anesthetic drugs in effective doses may suppress brain excitability and epileptiform activity (Demetrescu & Julien, 1974).

Dahl, Gjerstad, and Skrede (1972) essentially reproduced in a cat the destruction inflicted by Velasco and Lindsley (1965) on the orbitofrontal cortex, but they did not succeed in eliminating spindles. In cases where the amplitude and stability of spindles decreased, there was a simultaneous decrease in the amplitude of the evoked potential produced by stimulation of the contralateral ulnar nerve. Dahl *et al.* maintained that the suppression of synchronized activity following a trauma of the frontal cortex could be a consequence of several factors: the disturbance of the hemodynamics in the cortex and thalamus (including the specific thalamic nuclei), the development of an edema, a lesion of the olfactory bulb, or the release of the reticular activating system.

These contradictory findings prompt one to examine the assumption that the leading role in the organization of S–W discharges may be played by the mesencephalic reticular formation (Weir, 1964). Lesions of the thalamus have a far less devastating effect on consciousness than do those of the mesencephalon; the field of S–W discharges induced by stimulation of the massa intermedia is smaller than that resulting from mesencephalic stimulation. One of the most eminent experts on epilepsy, Ajmone-Marsan (1965), maintains that if the nonspecific system really has any relation to petit mal in humans, it is via its mesencephalic rather than its thalamic components.

This assumption seems to be supported by experimental data. Most authors were unable to obtain the S–W discharge by introducing into the nonspecific thalamic nuclei Metrazol (Gastaut & Hunter, 1950), strychnine (Cohn, 1949), aluminum cream (Kopeloff, Whittier, Pacella, & Kopeloff, 1950), and penicillin (Ralston & Ajmone-Marsan, 1956). Levin, Wyss, Scollo-Lavizzari, and Hess (1968) reported that in one case the introduction of a mixture of aluminum hydroxide and metallic cobalt (which partly damaged the cingulate cortex) into the intralaminar thalamus evoked a seizure resembling petit mal and was attended by complexes resembling the S–W complex. However, it proved impossible to reproduce the effect.

The introduction of the drugs listed into the mesencephalic part of the reticular formation has furnished few results. Only Guerrero-Figueroa, Barros, de Balbian Vebster, and Heath (1963a), working with kittens about 1 month old, succeeded in reproducing discharges of the S–W type by introducing aluminum oxide into the thalamus and the mesencephalic reticular formation. The time between lesion and onset of the S–W discharge in this study appeared to be correlated with the age of the animal at the time of alumina implantation. Younger animals developed the S–W pattern as early as several hours after implantation; in animals about 30 days old the latency of abnormal activity onset was as long as several days. In association with the S–W pattern the animals exhibited generalized diminution of muscle tone, intermittent facial contractions, and slowed breathing or respiratory arrest.

Careful inspection of the illustrations of the paper revealed one distinctive feature of this model: S–W discharges were very prominent in subcortical regions (mainly in the thalamus and the mesencephalic reticular formation), but they were far less evident in some cortical leads and sometimes even absent in the cortex (Guerrero-Figueroa *et al.*, Figures 3, 4, and 6). It is rather strange that in the presence of such strong activity in the centrencephalon, no generalized and bisynchronous S—W activity was seen in the cortex. At best this model does not support the idea that "a petit mal has its focus of irritation in the higher brain stem [Penfield, 1969, p. 800] ."

On the other hand, Starzl, Neimer, Dell, and Forgrave (1953) proved that, in the case of convulsive activity induced by Metrazol injection, the S—W discharges develop primarily in the cortex and spread to the subcortical nuclei—first to the specific, then to the associative, and finally to the intralaminar.

It was possible to obtain a potential similar in shape to the S—W discharge by stimulation of the mesencephalic reticular formation with 3-per-second brief trains of stimuli (Weir, 1964; Weir & Sie, 1966) and by combining tetanization (200 Hz) of the tegmental reticular formation with thalamic stimulation (Ingvar, 1955a). The threshold of S—W discharges was even lower than that resulting from stimulation of the thalamus (Weir, 1964).

Unlike thalamic stimulation, electrical pulses delivered to the reticular formation evoke clinical manifestations similar to those sometimes observed during petit mal: nystagmus, slowing of breathing, instantaneous arrest of movement, light fibrillation of the facial muscles, and so on. However, the local application to the cortex of some convulsants (Marcus & Watson, 1966; Mirsky, Bloch-Rojas, & McNarry, 1966) and the stimulation of the cingulate gyrus, putamen, caudate nucleus, and other structures evoke both clinical and electrographic changes similar to those observed during petit mal (Arushanian & Belozertsev, 1970; Buchwald, Hull, & Trachtenberg, 1967; Hassler & Dieckmann, 1967).

The caudate nucleus holds a special place in this respect. Akert and Andersson (1951) found that stimulating the caudate nucleus produced in animals a syndrome resembling sleep. Interest in this nucleus increased when Buchwald *et al.* (1967) showed that stimulation of the head of the caudate nucleus evoked a surface negative wave and that this wave coincided with the suppression of ongoing behavior and conditioned reflexes.

Petuchov (1968) produced spontaneous S—W discharges in cats after the introduction of a mixture of Nembutal (10 mg/kg) and chloralose (50 mg/kg). These discharges were of the typical S—W pattern—3 per second, sometimes 4 per second. Unlike thalamically induced S—W potentials, they predominated in occipital leads and then spread over all the cortex.

This rhythm was first recorded in the caudate nucleus. It appeared in the cortex in about the third stage of narcosis, 3—4 hr following the drug injection, while the first sign of the chloralose action in the caudate nucleus was recorded after 2—3 hr of narcosis. This is a rather strange delay for the caudate to be considered a pacemaker. During most of the spontaneous S—W activity in the cortex and caudate, thalamic leads showed 9—10-per-second spindles, which appeared to be unrelated to either cortical or caudate activity.

This line of research attempted to locate anatomical boundaries of the centrencephalon by looking for a pacemaker, but those structures investigated failed to meet even basic requirements for a S–W pacemaker. On the other hand, Ingvar's (1955b) experiments with the S–W discharges in cortical islets demonstrated that the activity of reticular structures may be a factor in suppressing S–W discharges in animal experiments and in clinical practice (Guerrero-Figueroa, Barros, de Balbian Vebster, & Heath, 1963b; Lennox, 1960).

I have previously noted that 3-Hz electrical stimulation of the mesencephalic ventromesial reticular formation generated an evoked rhythmical response of a spike–wave shape, predominantly in the most rostral areas of the pallium (Weir, 1964). Weir discovered an interesting effect from destruction of the rostral mesial pons in an effort to obtain a stable preparation with a low arousal level. Lowering the arousal reaction level facilitates the development of the S–W response in clinical and experimental studies. Weir rejected the use of general anesthetics, which have been previously used (Pollen *et al.*, 1963). He succeeded in observing the spontaneous emergence of paroxysmal and bilaterally synchronous S–W discharges. The appearance of these discharges was observed as a stable phenomenon in only two cats and the frequency of the epileptiform activity changed over a period of time from 4 to 1.5 per second. Still, this effect resembled previous episodic observations in which S–W activity emerged following destruction in the mesodiencephalic junction area (Hubel & Nauta, 1960) or after brain-stem section (Batsel, 1960).

Morrell and Baker (1961) observed similar phenomena. During a study of the effect of anticonvulsants on the dynamics of the secondary focus in cats, they also studied the effect of chlorpromazine. It was chosen as a control drug for comparing the effects of anticonvulsants with those of agents possessing tranquilizing properties, which Weir (1964) later declined to use. It appeared that chlorpromazine tended to promote a transformation of the focal rhythm into a S–W discharge, especially when photic stimulation was applied.

Stevens, Nakamura, Milstein, Okuma, and Llinas (1964) made a systematic study of the changes of focal activity evoked by injection of a concentrated suspension of aluminum hydroxide into the visual cortex of cats. After the formation of an epileptic focus, additional destruction was effected in the midbrain tegmentum area. Cats having minor lesions in the medial and especially the lateral areas of the reticular formation developed paroxysmal discharges resembling S–W complexes. Some animals displayed an increased sensitivity to flicker, a feature typical of petit mal. This effect was not observed against a background of pure focal epilepsy and emerged only as the result of brain-stem damage.

Stevens *et al.* found that spike–wave hypersynchrony was not a consequence of sleep. Although the animals were initially less active, partly because of the presence of serious neurological defects, normal alertness returned 24–48 hr after surgery, but S–W discharges continued to appear in the EEG. In discussing these data the authors concluded that "in addition to 'centrencephalic epilepsy,' the term introduced by Penfield and Jasper to describe the seizure induced by epileptogenic discharge originating in the central integratory system of the higher brain-stem and thalamus, it appears that occurrence of similar discharges is also favored by a 'centrasthenic' effect [1974, p. 474]."

If we assume that petit mal epilepsy is generally associated with a cortical lesion, the study of Stevens *et al.* may be considered an important breakthrough, increasing our understanding of the manner in which the generalized epileptiform rhythm develops from focal activity. However, we cannot at this stage conclude that petit mal is always associated with a focal lesion. Some experimental research suggests that lesions in the reticular activating system are sufficient to produce S–W reorganization of EEG activity (Batsel, 1960; Hubel & Nauta, 1960).

Milhorat, Baldwin, and Hantman (1966) pursued this line of research. They subjected rhesus monkeys to enucleation of the thalamus or hemisection of the midbrain tegmentum. These lesions were created singly or in combination with split brain lesions. Following the unilateral lesion of the projections of the reticular formation at the mesencephalic or diencephalic level, synchronization of the EEG and a lowering of convulsive thresholds occurred in the homolateral hemisphere. Damage to the homolateral hemisphere, as well as to the crossed rostral reticular pathways, led to a further intensification of synchronization and a further lowering of thresholds for epileptiform activity. Myoclonus, which formerly could be provoked by the introduction of Metrazol, now emerged spontaneously. Milhorat *et al.* concluded that the reticular formation satisfies the criteria for a centrencephalic system, and that this area of the brain is essential for the organization of epilepsy. They added that they believed the reticular system exerted this influence passively, meaning that "it operates by yielding inhibitory control rather than by actively elaborating the epileptiform discharge [1966, p. 610]." Nevertheless, the effect of destruction in the area of the centrencephalon may simply be a nonspecific consequence of a serious brain lesion. Indeed, the data in the study illustrate that on the fifth and tenth day after surgery, acute phenomena of irritation prevail and epileptiform activity of various origins is registered. Judging from the configuration of the discharges, only the complexes given in Figure 1 of the paper cited display some similarity with W–S-type discharges. There is no apparent similarity even in the subsequent illustrations given by Milhorat *et al.* (1966). Since the authors give no criteria by which the S–W discharge can be distinguished from complexes similar in form but different in origin, the relation of this important study to an understanding of the mechanisms of petit mal remains doubtful.

Marcus and Watson (1966) challenged the centrencephalic theory by stressing the importance of the corpus callosum in bilateral synchronization of the seizure discharges. Discharges were produced by bilateral application of filter paper tabs soaked with 0.5–1% strychnine sulfate, 1–2% estrogenic conjugated substances, or 10% Metrazol. In intact artificially ventilated cats the spikes, waves, or 2–4-Hz spike–waves appeared to be bilaterally synchronized within 0–12 msec. They were already synchronous prior to the appearance of seizure activity in medial thalamic nuclei. Complete section of the corpus callosum disrupted this synchrony.

Practically the same pattern was recorded in bilaterally isolated blocks of cortex connected only by callosal fibers (bilateral synchrony within 2–20 msec) and in adiencephalic preparations (i.e., following ablation of the entire thalamus, rostral mesencephalon, and dorsal hippocampus).

Although the evidence is very convincing for a transcallosal mechanism responsible for the bilateral synchrony of epileptic discharges of various patterns, it is far less clear whether a similar mechanism is operative for S–W complexes. Seizure potentials resembling the S–W pattern may be evoked in isolated cortical tissue, as was shown by Ingvar (1955b), and even in tissue culture (Crain, 1966). But the question arises whether they are really of the same origin as human S–W activity. There is little doubt that the discharges described by Marcus and Watson (1966) are more or less comparable to grand mal seizure patterns. The discharges shown in Figure 3A and Figure 6 of the paper of Marcus and Watson are simply a fragment of the self-sustained grand mal after discharge. Discharges shown in Figures 4 and 5 have a rather distorted form, which is not characteristic of the classical S–W pattern.

An abrupt onset and abrupt cessation of abnormal activity is a typical feature of petit mal discharges. It was the intent of Marcus and Watson to demonstrate this phenomenon in Figure 8, but the EEG record was taken without initial and final portions of the seizure. Even if they were visible one could argue that bursts of high-voltage activity interrupted by silent periods are a consequence of the isolation procedure. Indeed this case is illustrated in the other figure by Marcus and Watson (1966, Figure 5).

For these reasons theoretical implications derived from the transcallosal model cannot successfully compete with the centrencephalic theory of petit mal epilepsy.

It seems that all theoretically possible approaches to an experimental analysis of S–W discharges have been made. It is vexing that their results have been mostly inconclusive, indicating, as it were, that everybody was right in some things and wrong in others.

Similar difficulties are encountered in clinicophysiological experiments. Although a clinical absence is always accompanied by S–W discharges in the EEG, their presence does not necessarily indicate that a person really suffers from petit mal seizures or from epilepsy in general. Frequently, S–W-type discharges are registered during grand mal or focal seizures. Moreover, similar discharges in the form of episodes have been observed in individuals who have no epilepsy in their personal or family histories and who are suffering from other diseases.

These discharges have been found in depressive psychosis, schizophrenia (Fois, Rosenberg, & Gibbs, 1955; Hill, 1952; Rogina & Serafetinides, 1962), neuroses (Gibson & Kennedy, 1960), cerebral dissynnergy (Christophe & Rémond, 1951), lesions (Churchill, 1959; Lundervold, Henriksen, & Fegersten, 1959) and brain tumors of practically any localization (Madsen & Bray, 1966), migraine, mental fatigue, vascular disorders, and various organic diseases of the brain (Gibberd, 1966; Glasser & Hoefer, 1950). "Typical" absences and 3-per-second S–W rhythms have been seen against backgrounds of coarse diffuse and local organic process, including hereditary degenerative brain pathology (Andermann, 1967).

The divergence of clinical and electroencephalographic phenomena casts doubt on the diagnostic potential of the EEG, but these discrepancies undoubtedly are highly relevant to an understanding of the essence and dynamics of the epileptic process itself. The instances of S–W rhythm not associated with centrencephalic seizure exceed the frequency of occasional events and require special consideration. There may be several types of S–W discharge. Even for petit mal epilepsy one may find justification for treating every case of 3-per-second S–W discharge separately. Indeed, there is a tendency to identify classical S–W discharges and to evaluate them separately from "false" discharges. The latter category includes generalized discharges containing a rapid and a slow wave, focal S–W potentials, and generalized discharges emerging in short fragments only in response to activation (Gastaut, 1968). These distinctions are of diagnostic importance and are highly justified in a general consideration of the problem in its neuro-physiological aspect. We have at this time no satisfactory clinical, biophysical, or pharmacological methods for a delimitation of subtypes of petit mal epilepsy (Charlton & Yahr, 1967). It is important to consider the general cause of S–W reorganization (if one exists) and then to resort to an analysis of subtypes.

Another problem in the analysis of S–W discharges is the limitation of the current state of clinical electroencephalography, which makes it impossible to establish definitive criteria. Current techniques of analysis are ultimately biased by theoretical preferences. Stewart and Dreifuss (1967) described this situation as a paradox, noting in their article that it is as reasonable to attribute epilepsy to an undemonstrated cortical lesion as a nondemonstrable brain-stem lesion. However, when a focus in the cortex is discovered, generalization and bilateral synchronization of discharges are generally attributed to secondary recruitment (Penfield & Jasper, 1954) of a centrencephalic pacemaker by corticofugal impulses sent from the epileptic focus. Secondary synchronization of the cen-trencephalic pacemaker is believed theoretically possible; it is also thought to be one of the elements of the pathogenesis in generalized epilepsy. There are, however, no completely reliable electroencephalographic indices of such recruit-ment, and it is postulated simple from the alleged function of the oral pole of the brain stem. When discussing contradictory results it is still accepted to introduce a "correction" for the peculiar generalizing properties of the nonspecific system when S–W discharges are found in focal epilepsy. Now this traditional assumption, too, is being examined with the new EEG technology for registration of subcortical potentials.

It should be kept in mind that the exclusive significance of the study of the electrosubcorticogram in humans was supported by the widespread conviction among clinicians and a number of neurophysiologists that petit mal is an exclusively human pathology. Experimental models of the S–W discharge were believed to bear only a remote resemblance to the "genuine" potentials of petit mal. It was anticipated that many problems posed by the centrencephalic theory would be easily solved with the use of stereoelectroencephalographic techniques. Particular questions to be addressed were whether during petit mal there is a focus of "endemic" paroxysmal activity in the diencephalon; what temporal relations exist between cortical discharges during petit mal; and whether they can be controlled with destructions in the diencephalic area (Spiegel, Wycis, & Reyes, 1951). However, currently it has been impossible to obtain unambiguous answers to these questions.

There is a growing body of evidence that points to the ability of the cortex to organize and to pace S–W rhythm. Goldring (1972) demonstrated that the prefrontal cortex plays an important role in the organization of generalized seizures. Several of his patients formerly suffered from seizures of different types (including petit mal) and therefore the EEGs of some of them displayed complexes of the S–W type. Epileptiform discharges were first registered in the prefrontal cortex, then embraced the other sectors. Only after that did the convulsive discharge spread to the mesial thalamus. Convulsive discharges of the grand mal type caused by Metrazol also started in the prefrontal area. It proved impossible to evoke epileptic activity by 3-Hz electrical stimulation of the nonspecific structures of the thalamus.

Bancaud, Talairach, Morel, Bresson, Bonis, Geier, Hemon, and Buser (1974) reported, on the basis of their study of 10 patients suffering from generalized spontaneous seizures, that 3-Hz electrical stimulation of the mesial frontal cortex evoked electroclinical effects characterized as simple or complex absences accompanied by full or subclinical discharges of the S–W type. As the frequency of stimulation approached that of the spontaneous discharges the threshold of electroclinical seizure lowered. High-frequency stimulation provoked only tonicoclonic discharges.

Bancaud *et al.* therefore concluded that the cortex, notably the cortex of the frontal areas, plays the dominant role in the organization of generalized seizures. It has been shown that S–W discharges can emerge simultaneously in the cortex, in the structures of the limbic system, and in one or virtually all thalamic nuclei (Walker & Marshall, 1961, 1964).

It is interesting to note that Jasper (1949) warned that the S–W is essentially a cortical process that develops in response to thalamic impulsion and that this hardly warrants the search for a similar rhythm in the thalamus itself. This does not provide much support for the arguments favoring the centrencephalic theory. If the mechanism responsible for cortical S–W discharges is not to be found in the rhythm of a pacemaker, it is logical to expect at least an abnormal reorganization of the pacemaker's activity. "The activity of the apparatus constantly engaged in pacing rhythms must predominantly be rhythmic most of the time [Uchtomsky, 1938]." Yet, paroxysmal discharges of the S–W or other types may be absent in the thalamus during petit mal seizures (Hayne, Belinson, & Gibbs, 1949). They may emerge in any area of the brain, but the thalamus is rarely that area (Goldring, 1972; Niedermeyer, Laws, & Walker, 1969; and others). Even when discharges did appear first and foremost in the thalamus, there were not necessarily any on the cortical level (Proctor, Prince, & Morrel, 1966; Wycis, Lee, & Spiegel, 1949).

Angeleri, Ferro-Milone, and Parigi (1964) did not discover regular epileptic activity in the thalamic nuclei during S–W cortical rhythm. If the thalamus did show paroxysmal rhythms, they emerged later than those in the neocortex and were of a different frequency. The same is true of the basal ganglia, except that in this area epileptic activity was registered in even fewer cases. Contrariwise, structures such as the hippocampus and amygdala displayed minimal convulsive thresholds, and convulsive reaction was observed in them earlier than in other brain areas. In cases of centrencephalic epilepsy convulsive discharges in the hippocampus and amygdala were not only more noticeable but were also frequently the only serious electrographic disturbances preceding all others. In two cases spontaneous and evoked discharges of the 3-per-second S–W type were most clearly expressed in the rhinencephalic structures. These discharges frequently began before similar discharges appeared in the thalamoelectrogram or the EEG. In myoclonic petit mal epilepsy a burst of symmetrical spikes and S–W complexes in the frontal areas of the brain was practically always preceded by a series of rapid spikes in the hippocampus and amygdala, sometimes with an interval of several seconds. These patterns emerged in the thalamus considerably later (if at all) and were distinguished by lower frequency and amplitude. As a result, Angeleri *et al.* (1964) maintained that structures of the amygdalohippocampal circle play the principal role in the organization and maintenance of activity of a centrencephalic type.

The study of the subcortical activity of the brain in epilepsy has so far failed to provide strong support for the centrencephalic theory and suggests that many other brain structures could justifiably be considered S–W rhythm pacemakers. However, such a conclusion is *not* warranted; there have been no attempts to determine to what extent paroxysmal rhythms, obtained experimentally or encountered in the clinic, can be considered identical or similar to petit mal potentials. Indeed, S–W discharges of the intact brain have never been compared with identical (or seemingly identical) convulsive complexes in neurally isolated structures. Therefore, research to date cannot be considered conclusive, especially since some of the models of the S–W potential have little in common with the potentials of petit mal epilepsy.

Let me note here that the discharge I have consistently called spike–wave (S–W) is just as frequently encountered under the name *wave–spike* (W–S). I have until now intentionally ignored this difference in terminology, but the distinction in meaning is substantial. Unfortunately these terms are used very arbitrarily in literature.

The most pronounced component of the petit mal complex is the wave; the spike may be expressed weakly or not at all. Contrariwise, the spike is the dominating component of the discharge in focal epilepsy, and the wave following it is longer in duration and smaller in amplitude.

After inspection of the data one may suspect that in a great number of studies the S–W has been analyzed but the conclusions have been related to the W–S complex and the problem of the subcortical rhythm pacemaker, and correspondingly to the origin of petit mal epilepsy.

In particular, Gastaut and Hunter (1950) have drawn the reader's attention to the difference between the seizure potentials evoked by direct cortical application of Metrazol and those evoked by intravenous injection. They described, in addition to morphological distinctions, the difference in the excitability of the cortex to both types of potentials during the passage of a slow negative wave. Jasper (1949), commenting on the report of Cohn (1949), noted that potentials externally resembling petit mal complexes can be induced in various ways. However, these potentials are less generalized than those of petit mal complexes, and their bilateral synchronization is disturbed after section of the corpus callosum. For instance, a burst of S–W activity that emerged as part of a convulsive afterdischarge in both hemispheres was confined to the side of stimulation after the section of the callosal fibers.

Thus, there is reason to believe that certain authors discussing the role of the subcortical pacemaker in the formation of the cortical discharges accompanying petit mal seizure (often with radical conclusions) may be referring to convulsive discharges of a different origin. Some may, indeed, be referring to potentials of the W–S type; others, probably to the S–W type.

Another important conclusion drawn from the research of Angeleri *et al.* (1964) is that repetitive EEG recordings of the same patient at different ages and in the course of treatment can "reveal" a focal process camouflaged by W–S discharges. Minor seizures may begin to disappear as a result of treatment, become less frequent, or be replaced by major seizures as the patient grows older. Strobos and Kavallinis (1968) indicated that in the course of treating patients who had centrencephalic discharges a clear focus was sometimes found, located predominantly in the temporal lobe. They noted that centrencephalic discharges can be suppressed but that the foci of neuronal irritation, especially in areas with low epileptogenic thresholds, may remain during the controlled or inactive phase of the process. That this phenomenon is widespread is indicated by data on the relative asymmetry of the S—W rhythm (Gibbs & Gibbs, 1952) and by the presence of focal disorders in cases of "pure" petit mal (Howell, 1955; Niedermeyer, 1965). Therefore, there must be some additional cause or set of conditions that determines the development of petit mal. The presence of such a common cause is strongly supported by the number of factors that sharply increase the probability of the development of petit mal:

1. Genetic factor (Metrakos & Metrakos, 1961).
2. Immaturity of the brain. Only 2.3% of all epilepsy cases can be related to genuine petit mal; however, in children it accounts for 6—12% (Livingston, Torres, Pauli, & Rider, 1965).
3. Probably some hormonal factors, indicated by the fact that petit mal is more frequently encountered in women than in men (Charlton & Yahr, 1967; Gibberd, 1966).
4. State of inhibition facilitating development of petit mal seizures (Lennox, 1960).
5. Inability to provoke a clinical and electrographic absence if the patient has not displayed one previously (Bancaud, Talairach, Bonis, Szikla, Morel, & Bordas-Ferrer, 1965).

SECONDARY EVOKED POTENTIALS AS A MODEL OF WAVE—SPIKE DISCHARGES

The difficulties researchers have experienced when analyzing genuine epilepsy are, I believe, largely due to the fact that there has been no reliable model of the W—S potential. The classical method makes it possible to obtain a reaction resembling the W—S only in the event of continuous rhythmical stimulation of the nonspecific structures. The potentials emerging in the composition of the convulsive afterdischarge evoked by direct pharmacological or electrical stimulation of the brain and by other methods, relate, perhaps, to the S—W rather than to the W—S type. In most successful models, petit mal appears to be a consequence of the combination of two factors—cortical dysrhythmia and dysfunction of the reticular activating system. The cause of cortical dysrhythmia in these models may have been a banal epileptic focus (Morrell & Baker, 1961; Stevens *et al.*, 1964) or the use of immature animals with an infantile cortical rhythm (Guerrero-Figueroa *et al.*, 1963a). The dysfunction of the reticular formation was obtained by its destruction (Stevens *et al.*, 1964), pharmacological inactivation (Morrell & Baker, 1961), or the creation in it of an irritative epileptic focus (Guerrero-Figueroa *et al.*, 1963a,b).

However, irritation and destruction are by no means equivalent phenomena. Besides, in all models the development of the W—S discharge was regarded as the appearance of a new pathological phenomenon. The only exception is a model of Jasper and Droogleever-Fortuyn (1947), which hints at a more promising approach, namely, the search for normal reactions capable of developing into pathological ones. However, as mentioned previously, the evolution of normal reactions into the pathological class could not be brought about.

Therefore, the further analysis of the pathogenesis of petit mal requires answers to three questions:

1. Are there normal precursors of convulsive discharges of the W–S type; is it possible to reproduce them in an animal experiment and to describe the conditions making the normal cerebral rhythm epileptic?
2. To what extent is the rostral part of the brain stem necessary for the formation and generalization of petit mal potentials?
3. What is the nature of 3-per-second W–S discharges emerging from a normal precursor?

Experimental discharges must satisfy certain requirements if the resulting data are to be considered relevant to the pathogenesis of petit mal:

1. The experimental discharges must coincide with genuine petit mal potentials in form, frequency localization, and duration of the burst.
2. They must emerge spontaneously and also be evoked by the same activating agents under the same conditions as in man.
3. They must be suppressed under the influence of the same factors under the same conditions as in man.
4. Appearance of experimental W–S rhythms in the EEGs of animals should be accompanied by either disturbance of consciousness or its complete loss for a duration comparable to that in man.

These are rather severe requirements. Therefore, at first I wanted only to see the transformation of some spontaneous or evoked components of the EEG into W–S discharges—for example, an evolution of the thalamic S–W evoked rhythmic response into a genuine W–S discharge. It would then be possible to pinpoint the precursors of pathologic activity, to describe their characteristics, and to deduce the neurophysiological mechanism of epileptization. However, probably because I was not hypnotized by the properties of the recruiting response, I saw in virtually every evoked reaction an S–W form. Indeed, the configuration of most cortical responses of a waking rabbit resemble, under certain conditions, the S–W pattern.

For the visual cortex (Figure 1-1), however, a stable slow negative wave of large amplitude following the primary evoked potential seems to be the most characteristic response to an adequate stimulus. It emerges immediately after the primary response to light or, to be more accurate, following the second

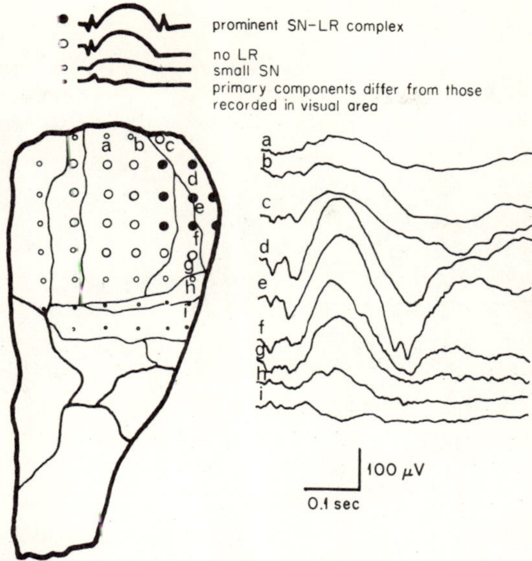

FIGURE 1-1. Typical configuration and distribution of the cortical potential evoked by a single flash. Unanesthetized semirestrained rabbit with needle electrodes; monocular stimulation. Here and in all subsequent figures, negativity of the active electrode is indicated by an upward deflection.

positivity (the time to the maximum of the latter is 55–60 msec), and after 150–200 msec it is completed by a *later response* (LR) in the primary visual area. The LR is in most cases represented by negative–positive–negative oscillations that are a direct continuation of the wave. In some cases, however, it resembles the primary response, differing only by its longer duration. It may also be multiple, i.e., consisting of two positive–negative deflections. Prominent LRs are usually recorded from the most lateral region of the occipital cortex, corresponding to the area 18 (Figure 1-1). Generally, the compound LR is followed by a repeated *slow negative wave* (SN). In a satiated, quiet, or dozing rabbit several such potentials are clearly visible. Hence, the slow negative wave–later response complex (SN–LR) is simply the first component of the sensory afterdischarge of the aftereffect (Ivanitsky & Myslobodsky, 1965).

While studying the nature of the LR we found that under chloralose narcosis or following the introduction of anticholinesterase substances, Metrazol, or chlorpromazine, the SN–LR complex was greatly increased and repeated sometimes as many as 10 or more times in response to a single stimulus (Ivanitsky & Myslobodsky, 1965; Myslobodsky, 1968b). This phenomenon was named the *exalted* or *wave–spike sensory afterdischarge* (EAD) (Figure 1-2). Spontaneously emerging bursts of activity of the same type were named *spontaneous equivalents of the exalted afterdischarge* (SEAD). Both are shown in Figure 1-2,

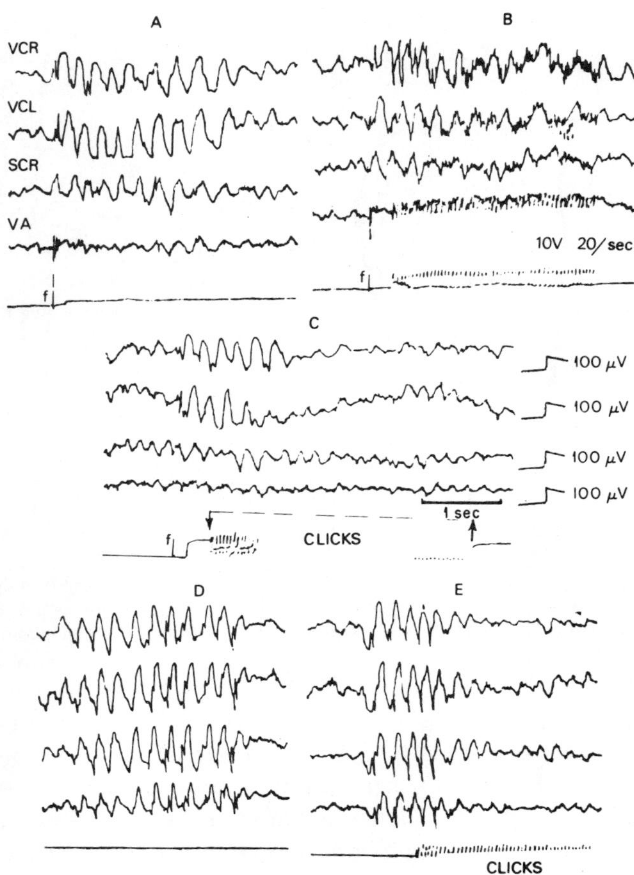

FIGURE 1-2. Wave–spike discharges, spontaneous and evoked by a single flash (f), after intravenous subconvulsive Metrazol injection. Unanesthetized semirestrained waking rabbit with chronically implanted electrodes. A, B, and C show EADs (exalted or wave–spike afterdischarges). D and E show SEADs (spontaneous wave–spike discharges, or spontaneous equivalents of the afterdischarge). VCR, right visual cortex; VCL, left visual cortex; SCR, right somatosensory cortex; VA, ventral anterior thalamic nucleus. Note the absence of wave–spike discharges in the VA and the suppression of discharges during intermittent click presentation (C,E) and tetanization of the subthalamus (B). To record W–S in the somato-sensory cortex and in the VA 13 mg/kg was injected, which for this rabbit was 4 mg/kg beyond the threshold level. With this dose W–S complexes acquired a multiple S–W pattern.

illustrating the picture of Metrazol poisoning. The SN–LR complexes making up the EAD and SEAD are morphologically identical with W–S discharges. They begin with a short negative–positive spike and pass through a longer positive–negative component (or a second similar spike) into the next SN. The duration of the spike (spikes) fluctuates within the limits of 20–60 msec; the duration of the SN ranges from 150 to 200–250 msec. Thus, the frequency of the EAD and SEAD coincides with that of the sensory aftereffect in a normal animal. This in turn corresponds to the frequency of the *sensory theta-rhythm,* the evoked variant of which is the sensory afterdischarge.[1]

Toward the end of a burst the frequency of the paroxysmal activity drops, sometimes to 4 per second, which is the lower limit of the frequency of the W–S rhythm evoked by Metrozol injection of the rabbit. Special measures must be taken to make it approach 2.5–3 per second. Even though this is a defect of the model, the search for measures to lower the frequency of this rhythm has made it possible, as will be shown later, to draw some conclusions about its nature.

Beyond the occipital and parietal cortex the SN–LR complex is only weakly expressed. To judge from Figures 1-1 and 1-2 it cannot be registered when the electrodes are located in the frontal lobes. In the map in Figure 1-1 the hemisphere is divided into four regions according to the composition of evoked potentials. Complex responses, including not only primary but also secondary SN–LR, are clearly restricted to the most lateral and caudal portion of the hemisphere, corresponding to areas 18 and 17. Responses with the SN but without the LR are recorded near the coronal suture. Rostral to it, however, mainly primary responses to the light stimulus are seen. Although the secondary complex is distributed over a comparatively extensive area, as a whole it should be related to the category of localized "specific" secondary potentials (Myslobodsky, 1966).

When Metrazol is injected this complex may be registered in the frontal lobes as well, but usually not farther than 3–4 mm rostral to the coronal suture. Correspondingly, both the EAD and the SEAD are observed in the rostral derivations—but only when an additional dose of Metrazol is injected, exceeding the dose necessary for the effect in the visual cortex (7–10 mg/kg). When Metrazol is injected slowly, W–S discharges evoked by photic stimuli develop first and foremost in the hemisphere contralateral to stimulation. Later they are registered in the symmetrical areas of the second hemisphere, and only after that do they spread in the rostral direction. With high doses the W–S discharges are somewhat distorted and acquire features resembling multiple S–W discharges (Figure 1-2). This is a period, however, close to the beginning of grand mal convulsions (usually doses exceeding 13–20 mg/kg).

When the electrodes are implanted in symmetrical points of the visual cortex of both hemispheres, a sufficiently high degree of synchronization of the EAD

[1] The sensory theta-rhythm should be distinguished from the hippocampal stress rhythm, which in rabbits and rats is easily registered from the surface of the cortex. The emergence of the hippocampal stress rhythm generally leads to suppression of the sensory theta-rhythm and to lowering of the amplitude, or even to complete blocking, of the SN–LR complex of the visual evoked potential. Some information on this rhythm is given in the concluding section of the book.

and SEAD components is revealed. The maximum time differences during spike development are within the range of 20–35 msec, the minimum within 3–5 msec. These magnitudes are also typical for bilaterally synchronous potentials of petit mal epilepsy. The causes for incomplete synchronization, even in the case of relatively precisely controlled electrical (Ingvar, 1955a) and chemical (Cesa-Bianchi, Mancia, & Mutani, 1967) stimulation of the thalamus, also have yet to be explained.

Furthermore, against the background of the SN of the hypersynchronous rhythm the primary response undergoes the same modifications as against the background of the similar component of a sensory evoked potential. This means that on the rising and falling stages of the SN the primary response has a minimal amplitude and may in some cases be suppressed completely. When the primary response is noticeable during the SN rise, its positive phase is practically not expressed at all and the negative component predominates. Contrariwise, following the peak of the SN when it begins to decrease, there is a steep increase in the primary response. However, in this case the positive component is greatly augmented and the negative phase is generally absent. This relation is shown in the graph in Figure 1-3.

The secondary SN–LR complex is very sensitive to the level of arousal. Nociceptive and strong sensory stimuli, as well as stimulation of the reticular formation, tend to decrease the SN, EAD, and SEAD and often eliminate them completely. Small wonder therefore that conditions of quiet wakefulness or inhibition of the reticular formation are optimal for the emergence of normal sensory aftereffects as well as for the W–S rhythm. For the same reasons sensory

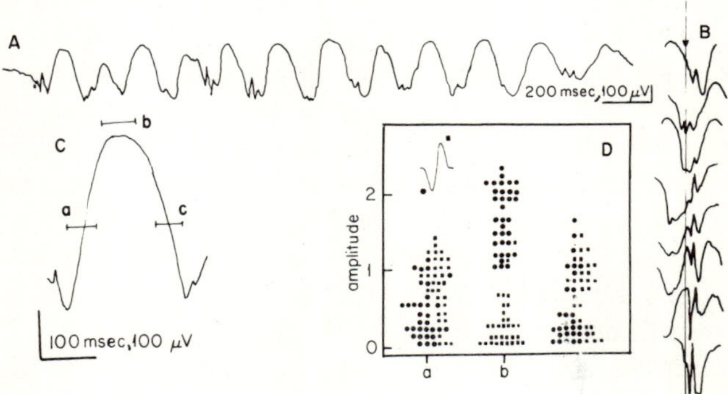

FIGURE 1-3. Peculiarities of the primary evoked potentials on different parts of the wave of W–S discharges. Unanesthetized semirestrained rabbit. A. Exalted afterdischarge to a single flash. B. Fragments of the wave with primary evoked potentials on its different parts (incidence of flash marked by vertical line). In D, arbitrary amplitudes are plotted of the positive and negative phases of the primary visual evoked potential developed on the three points of the wave shown in C. Accordingly, the abscissa shows points of the wave (a, b, c); the ordinate shows the amplitude of the positive (solid circle) and negative (solid square) components to their values in the period between discharges, accepted as a unit.

afterdischarges are rarely registered when the animal is rigidly held, even after careful application of Novocain to the pressure points of the stereotaxic instrument. Perhaps this explains why it is almost impossible to record experimental W–S discharges in a waking adult cat, which is a more aggressive, freedom-loving animal than the rabbit.

Metrazol-induced EADs and SEADs better resisted the action of wakening stimuli, and stronger stimuli had to be used for their suppression. A typical fragment of such an experiment is demonstrated in Figure 1-2. After the injection of 13.0 mg/kg of Metrazol, generalized EADs and SEADs emerged. Following the provocation of the EAD, some subcortical sites like the reticular formation of the midbrain, central gray matter, subthalamus, and hypothalamus were stimulated by pulses of rectangular current at a frequency of 20–100 Hz and an intensity sufficient for the development of the arousal reaction (Figure 1-2B). In other instances an intermittent click was switched on, whose intensity was also chosen to trigger the arousal response (Figure 1-2C). In both cases, during clicks as well as during electrical stimulation of the subthalamus, EAD suppression was observed. Parts C and E of Figure 1-3 show desynchronization of the W–S rhythm (SEAD) following the switching on of rhythmical clicks. A similar suppression of EADs and SEADs also occurred during tetanization of any of the areas mentioned or of the mesencephalon and diencephalon. It is interesting to note that despite the blocking effect of arousal stimuli, the Metrazol-induced W–S discharges were always preceded by a stage of desynchronization of the EEG. This was accompanied by behavioral symptoms of awakening and attempts by the rabbit to free itself from the holding clamps. This reaction was noted previously by Ingvar (1958). It is also known that in man W–S discharges are sometimes preceded by a short period of EEG desynchronization (Melnitchuk, 1971). I will return to this paradoxical effect later.

THE NATURE OF THE
SLOW NEGATIVITY–LATER RESPONSE COMPLEX

The sensory theta-rhythm in a rabbit and the derivative forms of evoked activity (SN–LR complexes, sensory afterdischarges) under the effect of Metrazol can evolve into a typical W–S-type rhythm. This does not exclude the existence of other precursors of W–S activity in the more rostral areas of the cortex, capable under certain conditions of bringing about the W–S-type rhythm. It was found, however, that it is somewhat easier to study the process of reorganization of the reactivity of the visual cortex. This experimental approach seemed promising, since the W–S complex in humans sometimes originates in the occipital cortex, especially in the case of photogenic epilepsy (Figures 3-3; 3-4). It was therefore found useful to make a more detailed study of the nature of the SN–LR of the visual cortex and to discuss its similarity with evoked complexes in other areas, including the potentials developed as a result of thalamic stimulation.

A series of experiments involving laminar analysis of electrocortical activity provided preliminary information about the nature of the experimental W–S. It was shown (Myslobodsky, 1970) that as the recording electrode penetrated deeper into cortical tissue, the SN amplitude became smaller. At depths of 0.8–0.9 mm the SN reverses its polarity. At approximately the same depth there is also a reversal of the primary potential as well as of the LR. With further penetration of the electrode, the deep-positive wave increases, reaching its maximum at a level of 1.2–2.0 mm below the cortical surface (Figure 1-4).

Thus, the generators of extracellular currents of the surface SN of the W–S discharge are located at approximately the same level as the generators of the surface positive components of the primary, and later reaction (the spike of the W–S discharges). According to the dipole theory several implications should be considered. First, the activity may be generated in the same cortical elements. Second, the dipoles should have a vertical orientation with respect to the surface of the cortex, which means that the most probable candidates are the pyramidal cells. Finally, the difference in the sign of the deep processes could mean that after initial excitation caused by a volley of afferent impulses there is long-

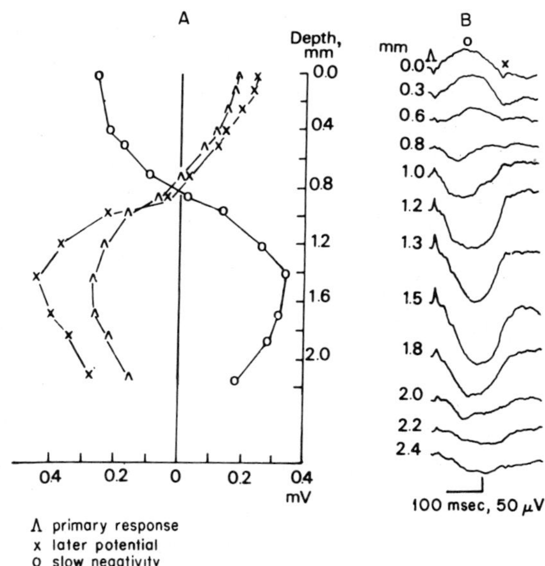

FIGURE 1-4. A. Amplitude of the positive phase of the primary response, later potential, and slow negativity plotted against recording depth in the rabbit's visual cortex. B. Corresponding tracings of averaged evoked potentials in different levels of the visual cortex. Unanesthetized restrained rabbit; monocular photic stimulation.

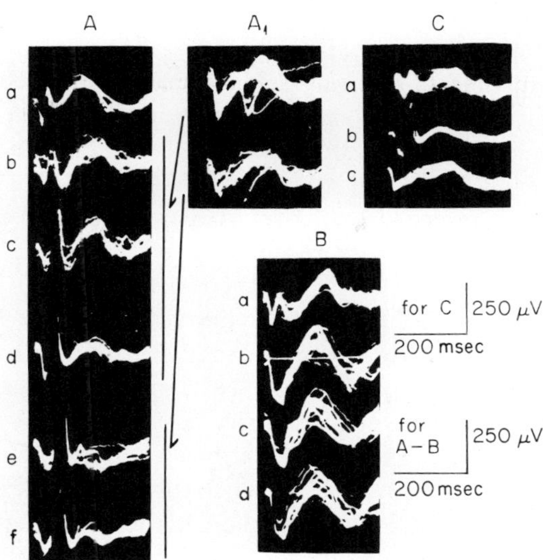

FIGURE 1-5. Sequential superimposed traces of visual evoked potentials recorded within several seconds after topical application of crystalline strychnine (A, A_1) and 3% GABA (B,C). Unanesthetized paralyzed rabbit, artificially ventilated. A. Strychnine effect: a, background evoked potential; b–f, different stages of poisoning. Note facilitation (b,c) and then suppression (d–f) of the SN. Increase of the photic stimulation frequency to 2–3 Hz led to the restoration of the SN (A_1). Arrows indicate the period (in A) when higher frequency of stimulation was applied. B. 3% GABA effect: a, background potential; b–d, responses taken every minute after GABA application. The horizontal line in b is the baseline control. C. 3% GABA applied 6 min (c) after the suppression of the SN by strychnine (b); a is the background response.

lasting inhibition, coinciding in time with the deep positivity (surface SN) and concluded perhaps by the repeated activation of the elements (LR).

Further analysis of the nature of the SN was made by neuropharmocological methods. Unfortunately, this approach did not provide conclusive results. But in order to maintain the coherence of this exposition, I will quote briefly the effects of the topical application of strychnine and γ-aminobutyric acid (GABA). The studies were made in acute experiments on unanesthetized (paralyzed) rabbits having an exposed cortex. The results of more than 30 experiments on 10 rabbits were coincident.

As Figure 1-5 shows, at an early stage of poisoning the topical application of strychnine intensifies the amplitude and prolongs the duration of the SN. But with the development of regular strychnine discharges the SN is gradually suppressed, concurrent with intensification of the spontaneous and evoked strychnine discharges (Figure 1-5A). Thus the final result of the strychnine effect coincides with the observations of Pollen and Sie (1964). These observations, too, can be explained by the ability of strychnine to block the process of postsynaptic inhibition (Pollen & Ajmone-Marsan, 1965; Stefanis & Jasper, 1965). This in turn is further evidence for the inhibitory nature of the SN.

It appears, however, that stimulation with 2–3 Hz light pulses immediately restores the SN of the visual evoked potential, VEP (Figure 1-5A$_1$). This restoration is due to the fact that the increase in frequency eliminates the strychnine discharge associated with the primary response and thus unmasks the SN. The amplitude of this unmasked SN at the stage of stable spontaneous activity of the focus is lower than initially; but its presence, as well as its marked intensification at the very beginning of strychnine poisoning, shows that the synaptic activities composing the SN are more complex than previously suspected.

Special studies (Myslobodsky, 1970a) showed that in rabbits up to 1 month of age (7–25 days) strychnine hardly ever suppresses the SN. It will be seen from Figure 1-6 that following the application of crystalline strychnine to the dural surface the SN of the evoked potential grows, its amplitude increases, and the LR is as marked as the primary response. When a second stimulus was applied

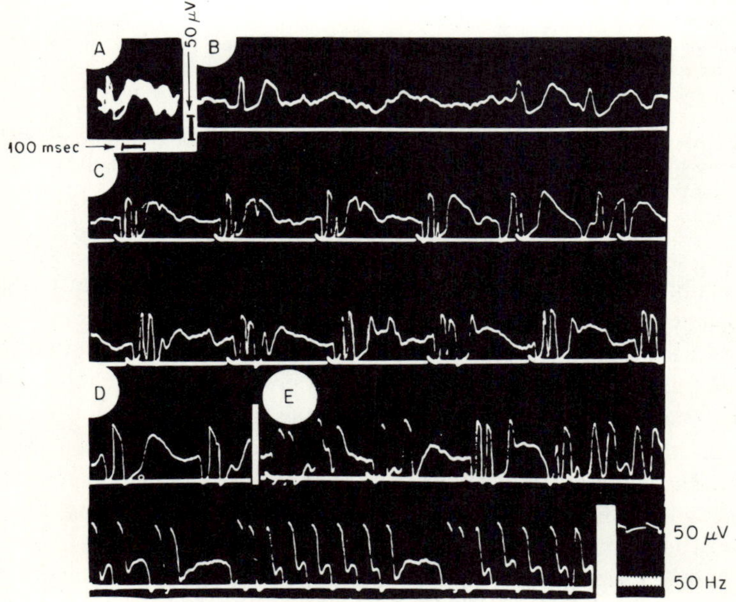

FIGURE 1-6. Effect of local strychnine application on the visual cortex of a rabbit 20 days after birth. Acute experiment (unanesthetized paralyzed animal, semistereotactic fixation). A. Superimposed tracing of evoked potential to a flash immediately after application of crystalline strychnine. B. Spontaneous S—W discharges in the strychnine focus. C. Spike—waves evoked by light flashes. D, E. Fragments of self-sustained seizure activity after the cessation of light presentation. Calibration marks: 100 msec, 50 µV (A) and 50 Hz, 50 µV (B-E).

directly after the first, mature as well as immature animals displayed no recovery of the reaction unless the second stimulus was delivered after the termination of the SN. The form of the spontaneous focal discharges was similar to that of the evoked response and both may be described as an association of spikes with a wave (Figure 1-6A, C, D). But again, analysis of the responsiveness of the cortex enveloped in focal seizures shows that the discharges emerging in the strychnine focus, though resembling the W—S complex, are organized according to different principles.

The effect of GABA was no less ambiguous. Figure 1-5B shows that a 3% solution of GABA resulted in about a 40–50% increase of the SN 1–2 min after application. This was in part only an apparent intensification, since it was accompanied by a steep increase in the positive phases of the primary and LR reactions and by a distortion of the negative phases of both potentials. However, in addition to the enlarged amplitude there was also an increase in the steepness of the SN rising slope, and this was in no way connected with changes of the parameters of adjacent components.

SN is virtually the only negative evoked reaction facilitated by GABA. Pollen and Sie (1964) linked this effect with deep hyperpolarization. This electro-genesis is unmasked by GABA's suppression of the postsynaptic potentials at the cortical surface. To accept this explanation it must be assumed that GABA possesses a nonspecific blocking action and that in the surface layers *inhibitory postsynaptic potentials* (IPSPs) that mask the effects of deep inhibitory electro-genesis prevail.

In Figure 1-5C it can be seen that GABA applied topically after local cortical strychninization leads to a suppression of spikes and restoration of the SN. Continuing the trend of thought followed by Pollen and Sie (1964), it can be concluded that GABA has "sharpened the dipole" of residual hyperpolarizing potentials. However, Pollen and Sie noted—and I too have observed—that the SN is not simply restored in these cases; frequently it exceeds the initial amplitude. This casts doubt on the hypothesis of the sharpened dipole, since it does not seem likely that the very few remaining hyperpolarizing synapses not blocked by strychnine could create a field more powerful than the one they create under normal conditions.

It is equally difficult to assume that the effect results from the restoration of the activity of deep inhibitory synapses when the rapid development of the effect is taken into account. GABA, unlike strychnine, is slow to penetrate the deep layers of the cortex. According to Guselnicov and Supin (1968) and my experience, at a depth of 1600–1800 μ the effect of GABA is seen only after 7–130 min. Though the foregoing experiments did not really clarify the nature of the SN and the LR, they did show that drastic changes are observed in the process under study when methods for creating focal activity are utilized. My results were therefore only applicable to focal cortical epilepsy. I also learned that it would be helpful to study the responsiveness of the cortex during different portions of the SN of spike–wave complexes, to try to differentiate W–S from S–W.

But let us return to the nature of the SN. More definite information can probably be gained from a study of the activity of single elements of the visual cortex. A series of experiments was performed for this purpose. Most of the experiments were made with waking rabbits held in a special semirestraining device. The microelectrode was introduced into the visual cortex through a trepanation opening 1.5–2.0 mm in diameter. Liquid agar (3%) was used to limit pulsation. In most cases a glass micropipette (outside tip diameter, 0.5–3 μ; resistance, 10–30 megohms) filled with a $3M$ potassium chloride solution was used. The reference electrode was placed above the frontal lobes. The signal was fed into a high impedance cathode follower preamplifier of the UBP1-02 type Biofizpribor amplifier.

The experimental program involved finding a stable unit, registering background firing (if expressed), registering the response to a single stimulus, studying the restoration cycle (stimulation with paired stimuli separated by varying intervals), and studying the response of cells to a rhythmical light stimulus with frequencies of 3, 5, 10, and 20 Hz. The duration of the flash was 50 msec, the energy 0.3–1.4 joules.

In all, 452 cells were registered (mostly extracellularly), of which 140 were selected for analysis in this chapter. It appeared that 41% of the registered elements did not respond to the light stimulus. But this does not mean that they did not participate in the general convulsive reaction of the cortex. Neither visual nor statistical analysis revealed changes in the nature of the activity of such cells in response to single stimuli. This was clearly evident because the elements reacting to light displayed quite characteristic responses.

The 140 elements could be divided into four major groups according to their response pattern. The first group consisted of cells responding only by initial discharge or discharges and having a latent period, on the order of 20 and/or 50–60 msec, coinciding in time with the development of the positive phases of the primary response (16.9%). The cells of the second type responded with initial inhibition, followed by a later discharge (19.3%), coinciding in time with the later positive response. The elements of the third group responded with both initial and later discharges, separated by a silent period (29.9%). Finally, the cells of the fourth group (33.9%) responded by general activation. They could have been related to the third group, but the period of silence was usually shorter, and firing appeared during inhibition with a probability exceeding .5.

Even though this subdivision of cells is in agreement with data obtained by other authors (Guselnicov & Supin, 1968; Kondrat'eva, 1964, 1970; Polyanski, 1966; and others), the classifications are actually arbitrary, based on the probability of a certain pattern. Also, the type of discharge could change with the application of paired stimuli or as a result of mechanical lesion evoking depolarization of the cell membrane.

Figure 1-7A shows a poststimulus time histogram, constructed on the basis of 504 responses from 98 elements of the visual cortex. It can be described as a reaction of the third type, i.e., initial discharge with a latent period on the order of 15 msec and a duration of up to 70 msec, subsequent termination of firing for 100–150 msec, and late discharges continuing from several msec to 100 msec. During the next 100–200 msec the activity of the cells returned to their initial level. This supports the idea that the deep-positive slow wave (surface SN) corresponds to the inhibition of firing, whereas the later response is linked with its renewal ("rebound"). As can be seen from the histogram, the later discharge is no less powerful than the primary discharge, which possibly testifies to the active nature of the depolarization on which the LR is based.

Decisive proof of the inhibitory nature of the SN was obtained from the intracellular registration of the activity of neurons of the visual cortex, which revealed a hyperpolarization whose duration exceeded 100 msec. It fitted fully the duration of the silent period of the cell during extracellular registration of

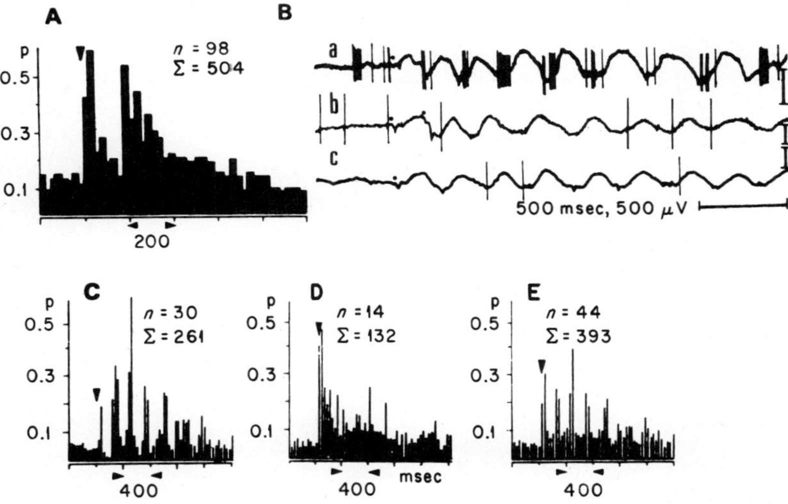

FIGURE 1-7. Correlation of the W–S afterdischarge and single cortical cell activity. Unanesthetized rabbits; area 18. A,C,D,E show averaged cellular response. Ordinate indicates the probability of cells' firing. Abscissa shows the epoch of the analysis in milliseconds. A. Poststimulus time histogram (PSTH) of normal undrugged cortical unit discharges. C–E. PSTH of cells after subconvulsive intravenous Metrazol injection. Incidence of flash is marked by an arrow. C. Cells actively participating in W–S discharges. D. Cells with limited participation in W–S. E. Summary PSTH of cells of both types. In B, the EEG response and extracellular unit activity (a,b,c) were recorded from the same microelectrode (incidence of flash stimulus indicated by dot). n represents number of cells; Σ represents number of reactions.

activity and appeared in response to the same stimuli—a flash of light, electric stimulation of the visual nerve, or visual radiation.

Skrebitsky and Voronin (1966) were probably the first to note that the duration of hyperpolarization of the cell membrane corresponds fairly accurately to the duration of the deep-positive slow wave (surface SN) of the visual evoked potential (VEP). The presence of a long-lasting polarization of the cell membrane interrupting primary *excitatory postsynaptic potentials* (EPSPs) in the visual cortex was also described by other authors (Fuster, Creutzfeldt, & Straschill, 1965; Watanabe, Konishi, & Creutzfeldt, 1966). It seems likely that the SN developing in various areas of the brain is based on a similar process. In any case, long-lasting hyperpolarization potentials were disclosed during the intracellular registration of cortical cell activity in response to stimulation of specific and nonspecific nuclei of the thalamus (Pollen, 1964; Purpura & Shofer, 1964), caudate nucleus (Hull, Buchwald, & Vieth, 1967), pyramidal tract, and cortical surface (Li & Chou 1962; Stefanis & Jasper, 1964). They were also found in the specific and nonspecific nuclei of the thalamus itself (Burke & Sefton, 1966a, b, c; Maekawa & Purpura, 1967; Purpura & Cohen, 1962; Purpura, McMurtry, & Malkawa, 1966), in the hippocampus (Spencer & Kandel, 1961), the basal nuclei, and other areas of the brain. Most researchers concur that these long-lasting polarizing potentials are genuine IPSPs, and it has been shown that they have all the requisite characteristics.

In the studies cited, certain assumptions were made about the organization of cortical inhibition. In this, all researchers naturally proceeded from basic data obtained from analysis of spinal inhibition. Thus if an intensification of the stimulus leads to an increase in the EPSPs' amplitude and probability of discharge of the given or adjacent cell, followed by an increase in amplitude and/or duration of the IPSPs, then the circuit of cortical inhibition may be organized according to the scheme of recurrent inhibition. In other words, it is assumed that the action potential proceeds into recurrent collaterals, which terminate on the given or adjacent cells directly or though one or more interneurons.

If inhibition is recurrent, any impulse activity of the element must be interrupted by prolonged polarizing waves. Indeed, such conditions are often seen in normal cells and are exaggerated by depolarization of the cell as a result of cell injury, when the intensification of its discharges at the end of the evoked pause leads to a repeated inhibitory period.

Another indirect proof of the presence of recurrent inhibition in the cortex can be seen from the restoration cycle of evoked potentials and cell discharges, i.e., changes of the secondary SN—LR complex evoked by the conditioning stimulus during the inhibitory period. This problem is to be discussed in a later section.

Stefanis and Jasper (1964) applied isolated stimulation to the pyramidal tract and showed that the IPSP develops in the motor cortex following an antidromic action potential (latency of 1.4 msec) with a latency of about 3.9 msec. During the registration of the summary evoked potential it was observed that the surface negative wave following the primary antidromic response is synchronous with the IPSPs (Humphrey, 1968).

Antidromic stimulation has the advantage of not only allowing identification of the excited elements but also giving an approximate idea of the organization of their synaptic activation in cases where antidromic spikes are followed by orthodromic discharges. The presence of the latter indicates that excitation, spreading antidromically along the axon, enters into its recurrent collaterals and orthodromically activates the same and other elements directly or via interneurons. Latencies of this magnitude for inhibition warrant the assumption that there are interneurons in the pathway along which the impulses are propagated. True, the data obtained on the visual cortex differed: Although the sequence of events in response to the stimulus was the same as that described previously, the EPSPs during stimulation of the optic tract (and antidromic spikes following stimulation of the fibers of the optic radiation) appeared only 1 msec prior to the IPSP. (Watanabe *et al.,* 1966). This time interval is more critical than in the motor cortex, a fact that made the authors doubt the presence of interneurons in this inhibitory circuit.

It should be borne in mind that interneurons have not yet been found in the cortex. They are apparently in the relay nuclei (Burke & Sefton, 1966b; Marco & Brown, 1966) and a thalamocortical inhibition path (Pollen, Reid, & Perot, 1964) might be assumed. However, the latent period of inhibition (at least in the visual cortex) is too short for such a pathway, and the interval between initial excitation and inhibition does not change whether the optic tract or optic radiation is stimulated (Watanabe *et al.,* 1966). Also, IPSPs are preserved in the cortex after its neuronal isolation (Creutzfeldt & Struck, 1962).

At a low amplitude of stimulating current the IPSP evoked by antidromic stimulation emerges in 83% of all cases without a preceding action potential (Stefanis & Jasper, 1964). In accordance with my data, up to 16.3% of the elements in the visual cortex react to a flash of light by an initial, long-lasting inhibition followed by a later discharge. Hence, activation of the given cell is not strictly necessary to bring about this inhibition. Inhibitory synaptic action embraces a large number of cortical pyramids, and the discharge of one of them, capable of activating the inhibitory cell, will evoke hyperpolarization along the entire territory of the given interneuron's "basin."

A comparison of the duration of inhibition affecting a single cell with the duration of the SN shows that the two coincide. During extracellular registration it is better to compare the latent period of the first action potential of the later discharge with the time elapsed before the later response (LR) reaches its peak. This shows that, with an increase of the LR latency, the latencies of the later cellular discharges invariably increase. This correlation is highly reliable. In addition to testifying to the connection of the SN with inhibition, this fact also throws light on the organization of inhibition. If the individual behavior of a unit is representative of the cell population behavior, reflected in the duration of the SN, and if some of the cells not responding with an initial discharge develop an inhibitory period, then the inhibitory synaptic action in the cortex is not only recurrent, but also mutual. As we shall see, this is of major importance for an understanding of the causes of activation, maintenance, and cessation of the hypersynchronous rhythm of the W–S type.

Thus, the structure of cortical activity during the experimental W–S discharge, evolved from the secondary complex of the evoked response to light, proved to be identical to that of the spike–waves of thalamic origin. In both cases the spike is associated with depolarization of most cortical cells, and the wave is associated with their long-lasting inhibition. Studies by Perot (1969) show that the same type of alternation of depolarized potentials with prolonged waves of post-synaptic hyperpolarization also forms the basis of S–W discharges in man. Indeed, when SN–LR evolves into SAD (sensory afterdischarge), an association of waves with inhibitory periods and spikes with cell discharges is clearly seen.

The EEG (a) in Figure 1-8A shows characteristic fragments of rather prominent SAD developed in a waking rabbit. In this case the female estrous animal was

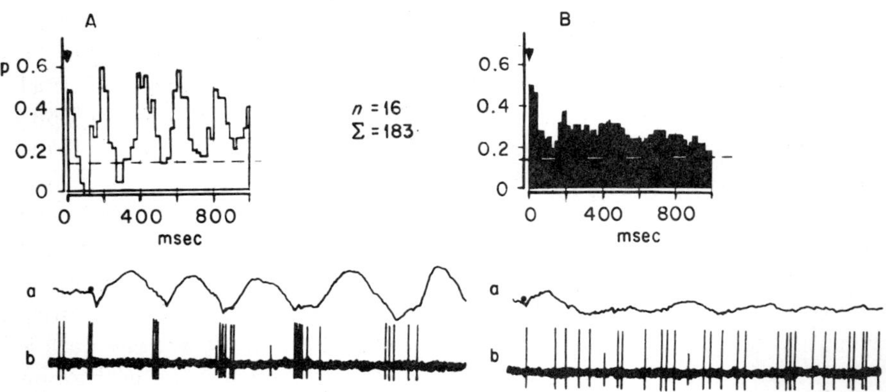

FIGURE 1-8. A fragment of EEG (a) and cell discharges (b) from the visual cortex of a female estrous rabbit during the stroking of the sacral region resulting in lordosis. In A, a flash presented on the background of synchronized EEG evoked SAD with group cell discharges corresponding to spike components in the EEG record. In B, suppression of SAD and desynchronization of the cellular discharges occurred after the presentation of sudden loud clicks. PSTHs of 16 cells show the consistency of this response in A and B. The interrupted horizontal line in A and in B indicates maximal probability of the prestimulus spiking level. Waking semirestrained rabbit. Arrow in histogram A marks onset of flash; in histogram B, onset of flash presented on the background of clicks.

used, since stroking of the sacral region during the estrous period elicits lordosis and easily quiets the animal. In other cases it is possible to attain the same results by simply habituating an animal to the experimental situation. Corresponding to each positive spike-like portion of the SAD, group discharges of the cells are seen (Figure 1-8A, a and b). The presentation of loud clicks desynchronizes cellular discharges and suppresses SAD (Figure 1-8B, a and b). Poststimulus time histograms of the 16 cells indicate that this is a typical pattern of correlation between cellular activity and EEG. It was assumed that in certain conditions SAD may be transformed into the typical W–S rhythm.

CELLULAR ACTIVITY DURING WAVE–SPIKE DISCHARGES

It has been established that the SN–LR complex is a universal response of the brain to a suprathreshold stimulus, registered in most areas of the cortex and subcortical formation in animals and probably also in man. In any case, it can now be said with a high degree of certainty that at least in the rabbit's brain the element from which the W–S process can be structured (under certain conditions) is "preformed."

The neurophysiological analysis of the SN–LR makes it clear that the probability of the emergence of a new inhibition–discharge cycle is determined by the later response, *rebound discharge,* of the elements. This view was taken by Pollen *et al.* (1964) to explain the emergence of repetitive W–S complexes, although in the study quoted reactivation of repetitive hypersynchronous activity was not observed.

It is clear that the frequency of the spontaneous and evoked oscillations must be inversely dependent on the duration of the inhibitory wave; the probability of the appearance of this wave increases with the firing of the elements. Eccles (1965) wrote: "Provided that inhibitory synaptic action generated by each burst response is distributed sufficiently widely to the thalamic neurons there is no need to postulate any phasing device other than the rhythmically generated IPSPs and a background excitatory synaptic activity [p. 94]."

This description of the pacemaker is obviously a general outline rather than a concrete explanation of the mechanism of oscillations in thalamic cells. Since practically all known rhythms are based on a similar phasing of IPSP discharges, this view does not explain the differences between a normal, stable synchronous or even hypersynchronous rhythmicity and that associated with loss of consciousness.

Normal undrugged cells of the visual cortex respond to a stimulus by a single inhibition-and-rebound firing cycle. Only a negligible number of cells go through a repeated cycle. Subconvulsive intravenous Metrazol injection rapidly changes this state of affairs, and the alternation of inhibition and rebound discharges repeats several times. In some units the number of repetitive bursts equals the number of W–S complexes in the EAD. Similar activity also accompanies the SEAD.

The activity of another 113 cells of the visual cortex was studied for analysis of this phenomenon. The cells can be conventionally divided into two groups, active and passive cells, according to their firing during Metrazol-evoked spontaneous and triggered W–S complexes. The active response is characterized by complete or partial suppression of impulse activity during the EAD and the SEAD (Figure 1-7B). Partial suppression is most typical and is manifested only during the SN; during spikes the cells emit discharges, frequently group discharges. Since the rapid components (spikes) may be complex, i.e., multiple, the cells can discharge during all their surface positive (deep negative) components. The record between two adjacent waves may be completely filled with discharges. The time of discharge is not closely related to the ordinal number of the W–S complex during the EAD and the SEAD, even for the same cell. Let us also note that between the types of unit activity during the W–S rhythm shown in Figure 1-7B (a, b, c) there is a multitude of transitional forms; cells may respond on some sections of hypersynchronous activity but not on others. Generally, most cells begin to discharge by the third or fourth W–S cycle, which can be seen in individual records and in poststimulation time histograms. It appears that cells fully terminating their activity during the EAD belong to the type that responds to light with only short latency discharges. Evidently the inhibition developing in these cases is so intense that in untreated cortex, as well as under conditions of Metrazol poisoning, the rebound firing of neighboring elements triggers repeated discharges of presumably common inhibitory interneurons. The elements are drawn into a new inhibitory cycle prior to the return of their membrane potential to its initial level.

Figure 1-7D illustrates a poststimulation histogram of the passive elements. These are cells in which the correlation between focal and impulse activity is either unstable or absent. They respond with an initial discharge and some tonic activation without a clear-cut inhibitory pause. This naturally is noticeable in a summary analysis but is difficult to distinguish in studying individual cell responses.

The poststimulation histogram of the *active* elements (Figure 1-7C) shows that six clear-cut inhibition–discharge cycles were registered during the analysis. Their number may be twice as high. The probability of discharges during the first rebound exceeds the probability of a short latency response to light, and the whole population responds with maximum and most regular activation at the end of the second or third inhibitory period. This is followed by a decrease in the probability of discharge and a shortening in the duration of each consecutive inhibition until inhibitions disappear completely. Judging from the high probability of discharge during the first rebound, the majority of the cells that faithfully follow the inhibition–rebound regimen must react to a single light stimulus with an initial inhibition and late activation. Or they could respond with two discharges, the first coinciding with the primary response and the second with the LR.

The foregoing description of cellular activity shows that some of the neurons of the visual area whose evoked reaction patterns to a single stimulus are of the inhibition–discharge or discharge–inhibition–discharge types relate to the group. Their number should also include cells fully terminating their activity. However, there are essential distinctions between the two groups, despite the presence of transitory forms.

From the former group one can distinguish some cells in which correlation with summary reactivity is high. These fire throughout the entire duration of paroxysmal rhythm. They apparently act as pacemakers for the other cells, drawing them into synchronous pulsation at different times. This may occur after the development of the first IPSP, which embraces a multitude of elements connected in parallel in the common inhibitory circuit. The following depolarization lowers their threshold to such an extent that they begin to discharge in response to asynchronous presynaptic impulses. There is a possibility that action potentials in recurrent collaterals activate the cells, functioning in recurrent excitation circuits, and that this promotes the emergence of repetitive discharges. These discharges are generated until the IPSP, evoked by the activity of the inhibitory interneurons, suppresses pulsation for the next 150–200 msec. At the end of the regular inhibition, a new depolarization takes place, and the cycle is renewed.

It could be expected that in time all elements whose thresholds have been exceeded by rebound discharges and which are synchronized by mutual inhibition will be drawn into a convulsive W–S rhythm. This does not happen, however; the EAD and the SEAD seldom last longer than 7–10 sec. Understandably, intensification of the reaction described involves the recruiting of new elements, but it is no less evident that this recruiting causes its own cessation. Considering the extensive spread of excitatory and inhibitory connections, even nonresponding elements are likely to display depolarizing or hyperpolarizing reactions (or both) in response to firing from the pacemaker cells. However, the amplitude and duration of these postsynaptic potentials are determined by the initial polarization of the cell membranes and many additional influences that converge on them in the circuits in which they are functioning. On the basis of concrete experimental data there are several possible behavior variants for such a cell:

1. The cell is drawn into the general ryhthm for several cycles, and the duration of inhibition coincides with its duration in other elements.
2. Recruitment takes place but the duration of inhibition differs from the IPSP of other cells.

3. The cell recruited is able to discharge but its contacts with inhibitory cells are limited and it reacts with a tonic firing.

The first case is obviously the most favorable for the maintenance of rhythm. In the second and third cases, 2–3 inhibition–discharge cycles with a phase shift from the basic rhythm may appear in the recruited cell. These discharges in turn may activate other elements and thus create a certain reserve, micropopulations of cells whose rhythmic activity differs in frequency from that of the spreading wave. At some stage they will interfere with the synchronous oscillation of the pacemaker cells, forcing their own rhythm, and the W–S activity will be suppressed. The validity of this conjecture for the W–S rhythm has been previously demonstrated (Myslobodsky, 1970a) on the basis of the theory of Andersen and Andersson (1968). It was concluded that with an increase in the number of cells united by a common rhythm, there is also an increase in cells whose IPSP duration differs essentially from the pacemaker-cell inhibitory waves. As more low-threshold elements are recruited into the common pulsation, there is an increase in the probability of a discord in that rhythm and of a desynchronization of convulsive activity. Hence, intensification of the W–S type of convulsive rhythm has a built-in mechanism for its termination, which is linked with the recruitment of new cells.

The preceding data indicate that the cortex possesses all the components necessary for structuring a convulsive rhythm under certain unfavorable circumstances. This conclusion is further warranted by the fact that in the rabbit W–S discharges result from the restructuring of the normal sensory theta-rhythm and not from a new process generated solely by an epileptic lesion in the nonspecific nuclei of the thalamus. But by the same token the sensory theta-rhythm and the W–S rhythm may be considered responses of the cortex to regular messages from the thalamus.

There is support for the view that the IPSP is the universal synchronizing mechanism of the brain, and parallel experimental and clinical data suggest that petit mal potentials can be organized without obvious signs of the electrographic participation of the centrencephalon. Together these ideas provide, it seems, grounds for a revision of the classical view about the role of a subcortical pacemaker, especially since the nonspecific thalamus was always advanced as the pretender to that role. However, there are a number of factors supporting thalamic involvement. Later discharges disappear in neurally isolated slabs of the cortex (Creutzfeldt & Struck, 1962), and the IPSP not only fails to grow weaker, but even intensifies. Also, the expression of the rebound phenomenon in the cortical elements is weak in response to their antidromic stimulation (Eccles, 1965) and the sharp cutoff of the anodal polarizing current (Pollen & Lux, 1966). Accordingly, the assumption was advanced that the later discharges of the cortical cells are of a subcortical origin (Eccles, 1965; Krnjević, Randić, & Straughan, 1964).

Since we are again returning to the problem of the subcortical pacemaker, let us consider ways of resolving the question experimentally.

EXPERIMENTAL WAVE–SPIKE COMPLEXES AND STRUCTURES OF THE CENTRENCEPHALIC SYSTEM

Let us begin with the technically simple procedure of Metrazol injection into various brain areas, utilizing the specific structure of blood circulation in the brain. The brain is supplied with blood from two sources: the internal carotid artery, forming the anterior part of the circle of Willis on the base of the brain, and the system of vertebral arteries, forming the posterior part. Blood carried by the carotid arteries supplies predominantly the cortex and basal ganglia. The vertebral arteries bring blood to the cerebellum and the entire brain stem and thalamus, including the midline nuclei. The frontal and lateral thalamic areas are supplied with blood from both sources. The connection between these two sources is insignificant and it is disregarded in clinical studies to determine the dominant hemisphere, localize epileptic lesions, and the like.

I have therefore attempted to use the method of intraarterial injection of Metrazol for the separate activation of the neocortex and brain-stem structures. If the assumption that the W–S rhythm may be organized exclusively in the cortex is true, this rhythm will appear sooner on the side of injection, for the threshold quantity required to provoke it will be attained sooner in the homolateral hemisphere. Metrazol injections were given in acute experiments in unanesthetized paralyzed and artificially ventilated rabbits having previously implanted electrodes. During the experiment the rabbit was held on its back in a restraining device. Under visual control a polyethylene cannula was introduced into the arteria subclavia to the right vertebral artery and fixed there. All other branches of the arteria subclavia were ligated.

Injection into the common carotid artery was simpler since it was only necessary to ligate the external carotid artery. In some experiments an artificial vessel was used for a loop anastomosing the carotid artery, which was convenient for drug injection and control of arterial pressure. This procedure requires more complicated surgery, and since it did not affect experimental results, it was finally abandoned.

Resting evoked potentials to light stimulus were recorded as a control before Metrazol injection was commenced. Later on, regular photic stimulation was used to check the time of the first EAD activation. Figure 1-9A shows that following intracarotid Metrazol injection the evoked W–S complexes (EAD) appeared first only on the side of the injection (a, b, and c). Metrazol injection was continued after the appearance of the EAD, and after some time a convulsive self-sustained afterdischarge, typical of grand mal epileptic seizures, appeared on the homolateral side (Figure 1-9A, c). On the opposite side the

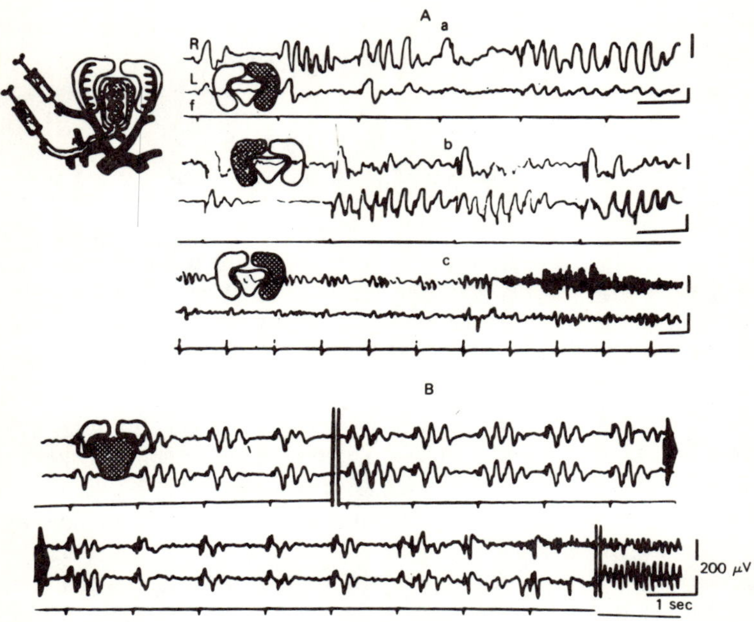

FIGURE 1-9. Effects of intraarterial Metrazol injection. Unanesthetized immobilized rabbit with implanted electrodes; acute experiment. A. Intracarotid injection (a,c: right carotid; b: left carotid). Note unilateral W–S development as well as unilateral electroclinical grand mal discharges in c, coinciding with W–S activity on the opposite side. B. Response to intravertebral injection (in accordance with the scheme in A). Two-phase action of Metrazol, i.e., activation and then suppression of W–S followed by grand mal pattern. Vertical lines denote intervals in records, for 1–3 sec. W–S in all cases evoked by rhythmic flash presentation. R: right visual cortex; L: left visual cortex; f: stimulus mark (flash).

concentration of Metrazol rose to a degree sufficient to activate the EAD, which coexisted with the convulsive afterdischarge of the homolateral hemisphere.

When Metrazol was injected into the vertebral artery, the EAD developed on both sides (Figure 1-9B). But this reaction is more complex and the bilateral W–S activation was only its initial phase. Further injection of the Metrazol not only failed to prolong the paroxysmal rhythm, but completely eliminated the temporarily developing hypersynchrony. It was replaced by the stable desynchronization of the EEG with a suppression of the SN–LR complex (Figure 1-9B). When Metrazol injection was continued during the period of the W–S rhythm suppression, the electrographic pattern of grand mal seizure appeared (Figure 1-9B).

Control experiments with normal saline solution in no case revealed changes in electrocortical activity. Other controls involving intraarterial injections of methylene blue and India ink showed that the Metrazol was selectively directed to different brain regions in accordance with McDonald and Potter's data for the rabbit (1951).

The last two stages of intravertebral Metrazol injection were very constant and always appeared in the sequence described. The first W–S stage was often missed since it was brief and always screened by the following arousal stage. Since nociceptive stimuli and tetanization of the reticular formation suppress hyper-synchronous activity, it is possible that in this instance, too, the EAD blockade is a consequence of a rise in the tonus of the mesencephalon's reticular structure. Indeed, the doses of Metrazol required to induce neocortical W–S by intra-carotid or intravertebral injection are practically identical. An arousal stage, however, never replaced the EAD before unilateral grand mal development in the case of intracarotid injection (Figure 1-9A, c). Thus, the first W–S stage evoked by the intravertebral drug injection may be a cortical phenomenon resulting from small amounts of drug reaching the occipital pole by way of the posterior cerebral artery.

During intravenous injection of Metrazol, W–S discharges are always preceded by a period of arousal. One had to consider the possibility that there may be two stages or two types of activation responses: the intravertebral-induced arousal that obstructs the development of W–S discharges or suppresses them, and the intravenous-induced desynchronization response that could promote the development of W–S complexes. In the latter case it would have to be assumed that the activation is a consequence of the "irritation" of the centrencephalic structures, the next stage of which is the organization within them of convulsive discharges. A W–S rhythm would be expected then to develop on the level of the cortex only after seizure afterdischarge had appeared in the pacemaker structures.

To check this assumption a special series of experiments was performed in 18 rabbits having electrodes implanted into different structures of the mesen-cephalon and diencephalon. The intent was to study the sequence of develop-ment of spontaneous and evoked W–S (EAD and SEAD) type discharges in the cortical and subcortical centers following intravenous injection of subconvulsive doses of Metrazol. These experiments were surprisingly homogeneous; in every case the hypersynchronous activity developed in the cortex long before any abnormalities appeared in the electrosubcorticogram as was shown also by Starzl *et al.* (1953). The only diencephalic structure registering hypersynchronous activity with a minimal latent period was the specific visual relay nucleus—the lateral geniculate body. The EAD and the SEAD emerged there simultaneously with or shortly following cortical discharges, but they never unambiguously preceded the neocortical W–S complexes.

Yet another fact provided a direct answer to the question about the role of the centrencephalic structures in the organization of the W–S-type rhythm. The emergence of the convulsive rhythm in nonspecific structures correlated with the disappearance of neocortical hypersynchronous discharges. (Figure 1-10 shows a fragment of a typical experiment in the lateral posterior thalamic nucleus and in the visual cortex.) This is particularly interesting because in 82% of the cases of suppression of cortical W–S discharges the development of seizure discharges was observed in the lateral posterior nucleus of the thalamus. It is precisely this structure that is considered an important part of the centrencephalic system (Van Straaten, 1962).

The very fact that the EAD can appear in one hemisphere only seems to cast doubt on the idea that its organization requires a pacemaker located in the nonspecific nuclei of the thalamus. However, another explanation of the unilateral activation of the epileptic rhythm can be postulated with equal justification. Such a pacemaker may exist in the oral part of the brain stem and its messages may be addressed constantly to both hemispheres; but the probability of the appearance of a paroxysmal rhythm depends in turn upon the excitability of the receiving structures. From the very beginning we deliberately

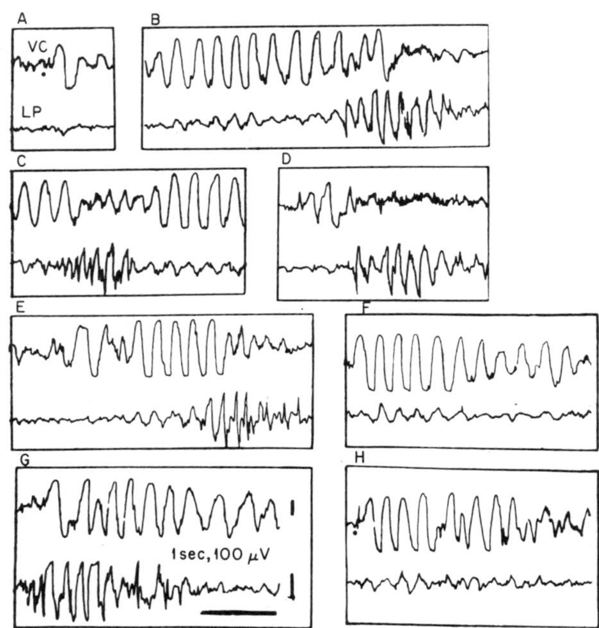

FIGURE 1-10. Interrelation of W–S activity in the visual cortex (VC) and homolateral lateral posterior thalamic nucleus (LP). Unanesthetized waking semirestrained rabbit with chronically implanted electrodes. A. Evoked potential in normal state. H. Evoked potential progressed into W–S afterdischarge with subconvulsive intravenous Metrazol injection. (Incidence of flash marked by dot.) B–G. Spontaneous W–S discharges. Note cessation of W–S in cortical leads after development of discharges in LP in most cases, except in G. Calibration noted in G applies to A-H.

ascribed a privileged position to one of the hemispheres by lowering the cortical cell threshold with an injection of convulsive agents. It is not improbable that we deceived ourselves by forming preconceptions about the results of the experiment.

True, this theory may be rejected on the basis of the data outlined earlier, notably because petit mal epilepsy rhythms first appear in the neocortex. Nonetheless, we were never firmly convinced that there was not an identical rhythm somewhere in the thalamus generated by cells at some distance from the electrode. That is why this assumption was subjected to thorough testing. We found that if preliminarily subthreshold Metrazol doses were injected into the carotid artery, followed by an intravenous or intravertebral injection of Metrazol, asymmetry of discharges was immediately recorded on the preliminarily activated side. This asymmetry is manifested in the sequence of EAD emergence, the number of W–S complexes, or the extent to which they are expressed.

The next step was the surgical removal of the rostral part of the brain stem in order to determine its significance for the organization of hypersynchronous discharges. The first experiments were made in acute conditions on artificially ventilated, unanesthetized rabbits. Under visual control effected with the aid of a binocular microscope most of the thalamus and other subcortical structures were removed by suction using the method described by Bignall, Imbert, and Buser (1966). The final interpretation of the results was based on data obtained in preparations in which the nonspecific thalamic nuclei, basal ganglia, hypothalamus, pulvinar, superior colliculi, and mesencephalic reticular formation had been successfully removed. A referential electrode implanted 1–1.5 mm medial to the lateral geniculate body (AP 5 plane) permitted accurate aspiration of borderline structures in the proximity of a dangerous region. The cavity inside the brain was filled with liquid agar (3%).

These preparations helped resolve many pressing neurophysiological problems. However, there is no doubt that this deliberately inflicted pathological state caused a serious disturbance of the hemodynamics of the brain. We were therefore fully aware that the postsurgical absence of activity of the EAD type, and even of the SN–LR complex, would not prove that the rostral part of the brain stem is necessary for organization of such potentials. But if it were still possible to register such activity despite these substantial injuries, the idea of a pacemaker in the rostral part of the brain stem would lose its attractiveness.

We obtained six successful preparations in which the evoked activity continued on the same level for not less than 4–6 hr (registration was begun 1–1.5 hr after surgery), and in which there was adequate aspiration of the central structures. Visual pathways were left intact. It was found that the sequence of events in response to light stimulus did not change. Following the primary reaction the same SN–LR complex developed, as before surgery, though its amplitude was paroxysmally increased and duration of the SN exceeded its preoperative values by 30%. During this abnormal facilitation of brain reactivity the episodes of W–S activity were recorded in the form of the EAD and the SAD, and their frequency diminished to 2.5–3 per second, i.e., to the frequency of the W–S discharges. For the first time we faced the possibility of fulfilling the very important requirement for a model of W–S activity.

Thus, in the undrugged animal it was possible to induce W–S activity simply by lesioning structures of the centrencephalic system and to see that evoked W–S discharges are no more than exaggerated sensory afterdischarges. However, at this stage of the study we could not confidently view the development of the W–S rhythm as a consequence of cortical isolation. We were reluctant to make such an assumption because of the coarse injury we had inflicted on the brain. But this experiment at least showed that the secondary SN–LR complex is a specific cortical phenomenon that depends upon the integrity of the visual pathways alone.

Later we refrained from such injurious surgery and the brain stem was destroyed in a prolonged acute experiment (Myslobodsky, 1968b). The structures of the oral pole of the brain stem were not subjected to aspiration, but were resected from one or two sides using the encephalotome, shown in Figure 1–11. It consists of a hollow rod, 1.5 mm in diameter, containing a movable stainless steel wire with a bent tip. By introducing the encephalotome along the midline through the corpus callosum, it was possible to cut the nonspecific nuclei of the thalamus, hypothalamus, and basal ganglia, and to carry out an additional section of the brain stem without damaging the cortex (Figure 1-12).

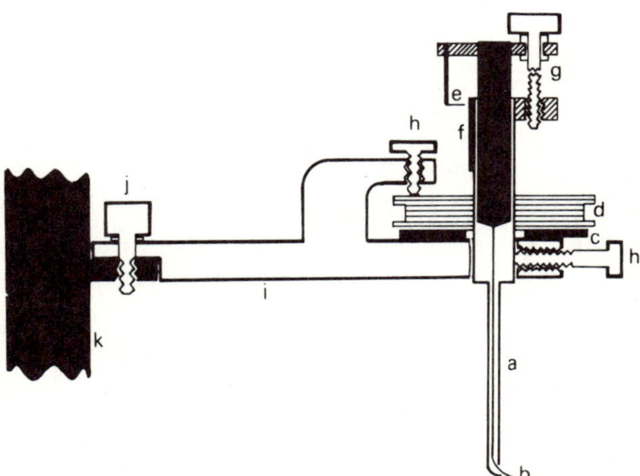

FIGURE 1-11. The encephalotome: a, cannula with cutting stylet; b, free end of the cutting stylet shown in working position; c, goniometer scale; d, disk with built-in pointer of angle of rotation of cannula; e, pointer showing free part of stylet with f, a scale of the length of the stylet; g, adjusting screw; h, screws locking the limb and the cannula; i, encephalotome holder; j, screw fastening the encephalotome to the stereotaxic device; and k, stereotaxic apparatus.

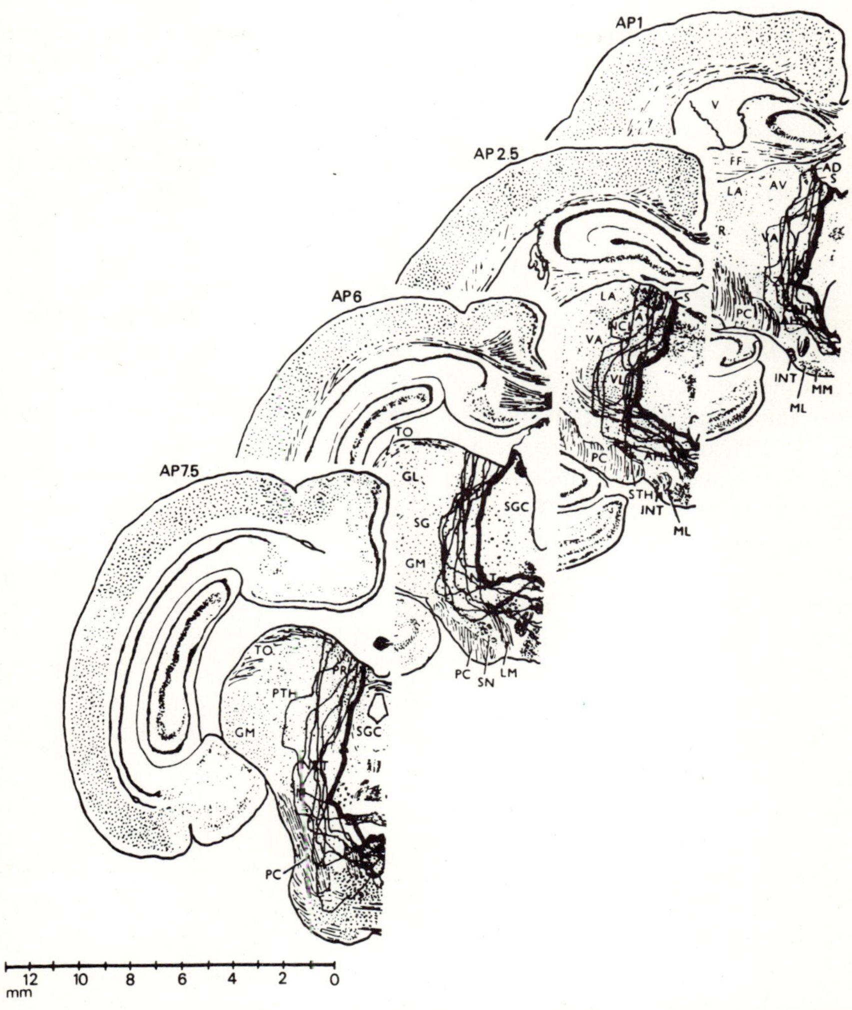

FIGURE 1-12. Reconstruction of lesions made with the encephalotome; superimposed on maps from Fifcova and Marsala (1967). Area of overlap shown by a heavy line demonstrates that main structures of the centrencephalon were lesioned in every preparation. AP, area preoptica; AV, nucleus antero-ventralis; GL(GM), corpus geniculatum laterale (mediale); LA, nucleus lateralis anterior; LM, lemniscus medialis; PC, pedunculus cerebri; PTH, nucleus posterior thalami; R, nucleus reticularis; SGS, stratum griseum centrale; STH, nucleus subthalamicus; SN, substancia nigra; TO, tractus opticus; VA, nucleus ventralis anterior; VL, nucleus ventralis lateralis.

Following extraction of the encephalotome, the bone defect was filled with liquid agar (3%) and then closed with a plastic film fixed with dental cement. We consider this experiment to be acute and expected the animals to be in a bad state. Yet, of the 19 animals on which we operated, 7 lived with bilateral, and 3 with unilateral, destructions of the oral brain stem (Figure 1-12). The others perished on the first or second day in a state of deep coma, aggravated by pneumonia and atony of the gastrointestinal tract. The rabbits that remained alive were mostly immobile, their pain thresholds were markedly heightened, and their escape reaction was virtually absent. Episodic myoclonic reaction often developed against this background.

Figure 1-13 shows that the spontaneous and evoked W–S rhythms are regular concomitants of the section of the thalamus and mesencephalon. During hemithalamotomy the EAD and the SEAD were expressed mainly in the homolateral hemisphere, though they were often registered on both sides. In cases when the lateral geniculate body was damaged no W–S rhythm originating from the SN–LR complex was registered at all. Thus, let me emphasize once more that paroxysmal discharges were the only consequence of the destruction of the higher-brain-stem structures. Their frequency was similar to that of genuine petit mal potentials, 2.5–3 per second. The slowing of the W–S discharges reflected postoperative changes in the secondary SN–LR complex of the visual evoked response. As shown in Figure 1-13A, there was a paroxysmal growth of the complex together with an increase in SN duration. The latter was of the same order as in aspiration experiments. The slightest changes in SN duration were correlated with immediate changes in the frequency of the W–S activity.

The other index pointing to the common origin of the evoked SN and the

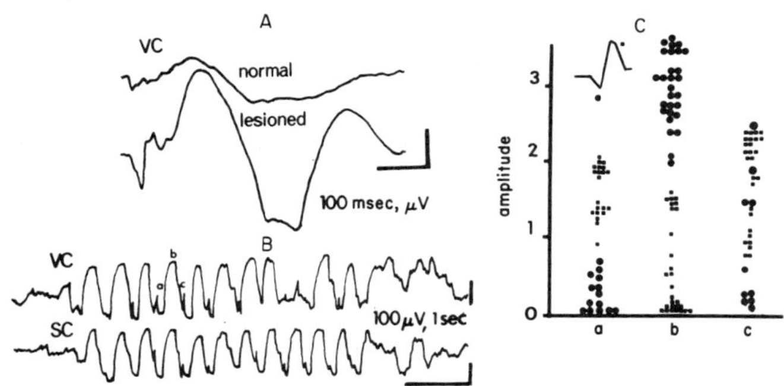

FIGURE 1-13. Facilitation of the amplitude and duration of the SN–LR complex and the development of 3-per-second W–S activity 4 days after lesion of the oral pole of the brain stem with the encephalotome. A. Averaged evoked potential to a single flash in the visual cortex (VC) in a semirestrained rabbit before and after the lesion. B. An example of spontaneous W–S activity in the visual and sensorimotor cortex (SC). C. Changes of the positive (solid circle) and negative (solid square) phase of the primary evoked potential on the three portions of the wave (a,b,c) shown in B. Compare with Figure 1-3.

wave of the seizure potential was provided by a comparison of cortical responsiveness during the development of both waves. It revealed that the modulation of the primary potential by the background wave was identical for a normal evoked SN or a seizure component. When photic stimuli were applied during selected portions of the seizure discharge (Figure 1-13C), it appeared that on the ascending and descending slopes of the wave there was a marked suppression of the primary response as demonstrated earlier in Figure 1-3D. If the response was of normal amplitude or even slightly facilitated, there were distinct changes in its configuration involving the predominance of its negative component. The positive phase of the primary responses developed on the top of the wave and the beginning of its descending slope was always paroxysmally augmented. Here the shape of the primary response changed due to the suppression of the negative component.[2]

The variant of the "prolonged acute experiment" thus fully justified itself. Again it appeared to be possible to receive an augmented evoked SN−LR complex and to reproduce W−S rhythms from lesions in the reticular−limbic system without additional injection of Metrazol. The drug was even superfluous in this case since 2−6 mg/kg was sufficient to activate grand mal seizure. This dose is 50% or 25% of that which induces electrocortical self-sustained seizure in unoperated animals. Another advantage of the method was that it allowed the study of both the outcome of severe injury to brain tissue and the establishment of new cortico−subcortical relations when the brain was given at least a slight chance for recovery.

At this stage of research it seemed justified to assume that the structures of the higher brain stem are not essential for the organization of convulsive activity of the W−S type. In fact, they even obstruct its emergence. This conclusion could also have been drawn when it was first noticed that the amplitude and probability of the emergence of W−S complexes is inversely dependent on the degree of activity of the desynchronizing structures of the reticular formation.

Let me, however, continue consideration of the role of the nonspecific system. The experiments just discussed have a vulnerable spot, which stems from the effectiveness of the operations in inducing the W−S rhythm. We were unable to establish which structures acted as stabilizers of the cerebral activity. In other words, we were unable to determine the removal of which nervous centers promoted the hypersynchronization of the electrocortical activity. Perhaps the answer to that question has already been found, but we consider it doubtful that

[2] Cortical responsiveness was examined here simply to identify seizure discharges and to test the degree of similarity of W−S complexes of different origin. The changes of the primary response against a background of evoked secondary SNs were perfectly identical. The details of the restoration of the primary potential on the background of the secondary negativity evoked by a preceding stimulus (i.e., recovery cycle) will be presented and discussed in a separate section (see Chapter 3).

so differentiated a system as the reticular—limbic complex should ensure the reliable and nonspecific maintenance of cerebral rhythmicity by acting according to a critical-mass principle. Indeed, one cannot exclude the possibility that the development of W—S discharges resulted from the lesion of some very definite structure that accidently appeared in the visual field of the encephalotome. If such a structure really exists, it is well worth analyzing the mechanisms controlling cortical activity in an attempt to discover it.

The areas for subsequent local destruction were chosen in accordance with preliminary experiments to select structures whose stimulation evoked maximal behavioral "thumping" and an electrographic arousal reaction that correlated with the blockade of synchronized activity and suppression of the SN—LR complex. Generally, dc anodes were used to destroy the tegmental and pontine reticular nuclei, central gray matter of the mesencephalon, superior colliculi, nonspecific nuclei of the thalamus, hypothalamic nuclei, and the subthalamus. In addition, the lateral geniculate body, pulvinar, and a number of other centers (septum, orbitofrontal cortex) were also destroyed, mainly for the purpose of control.

The selective destruction of the enumerated structures and damage to the epithalamus, notably the habenular nuclei and parts of the dorsal thalamus, lead to the appearance in the cortex of stable EAD and SEAD. The effect manifests itself predominantly on the side of the injury but may also be bisynchronous. These discharges do not differ from the W—S rhythm described previously and require no special description. However, I do wish to point out their great stability in the face of the action of awakening stimuli and tetanization of the mesencephalic reticular formation (see Figure 1-14). It is noteworthy that this is true while occasional desynchronization of the background rhythm can still be evoked.[3]

Ambiguous results were obtained when the subcortical visual centers were destroyed. Injuries in the regions of the pretectum, pulvinar, and superior colliculi did not eliminate the SN—LR complex but made it even more clearly expressed. They increased the duration of the SN, which resulted in a lowering of the hypersynchronous rhythm frequency when Metrazol was injected.

During destruction of the lateral geniculate body the EAD and the SEAD were partly or fully disorganized in the side of the injury. They did not emerge in the subcortical structures following Metrazol injection (Figure 1-15). Bilateral destruction of the lateral geniculate body suppressed the W—S discharges on both

---

[3] The impression is gained that there are two types of activation reaction. One is able to block hypersynchronous rhythm of the EAD and SEAD type, and the other is not. We have already encountered similar phenomena when analyzing the effects of intravenous and intraarterial injections of Metrazol. Their effects resemble those of d-amphetamine, suppressing SN—LR, and of the anticholinesterase substance halantamine, intensifying the SN—LR complex and evoking EAD. Both drugs are potent activators of EEG arousal.

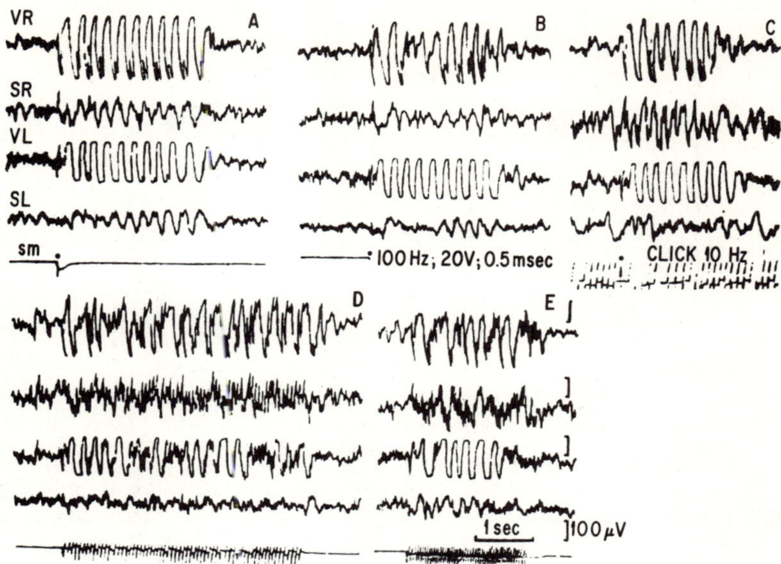

FIGURE 1-14. Photoconvulsive response in the visual cortex after right epithalamic lesion. A. Wave–spike afterdischarge to a single flash in resting state. B. Afterdischarge to a single flash evoked against a background of high-frequency electrical stimulation of the skin on the hindlimb of the animal. C. Wave–spike afterdischarge evoked during 10-Hz presentation of loud clicks. D, E. Wave–spikes during intermittent photic stimulation. Waking semirestrained rabbit 27 days after the operation. Chronically implanted electrodes over the right and the left visual (VR, VL) and somatosensory (SR, SL) cortex. Stimulus mark, sm. Single light stimuli also marked by a dot.

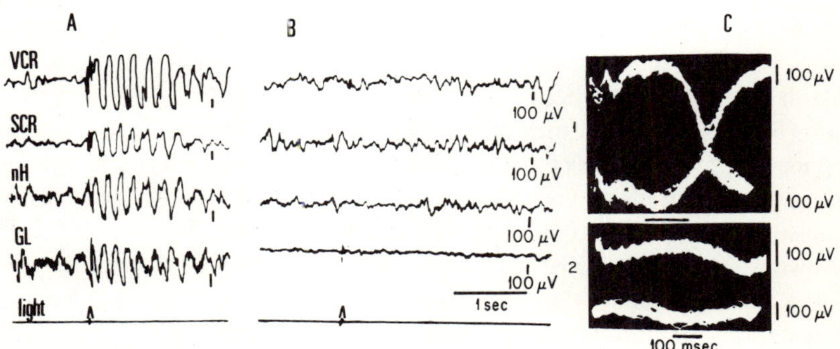

FIGURE 1-15. Elimination of wave–spike afterdischarge in cortical and subcortical areas after lesion in lateral geniculate nucleus. Semirestrained waking rabbit with chronically implanted electrodes 8 days after the lesion. A. Wave–spikes evoked by a single flash after intravenous 7.3 mg/kg Metrazol injection. B. Effect of the lesion tested on a background of Metrazol poisoning. C. Control records of superimposed evoked potentials of the visual cortex and the lateral geniculate nucleus before (1) and after (2) the lesion in the same rabbit. Flash was presented at the beginning of the trace. (VCR, right visual cortex; SCR, right sensorymotor cortex; nH, habenular nucleus; GL, lateral geniculate nucleus on the same side.)

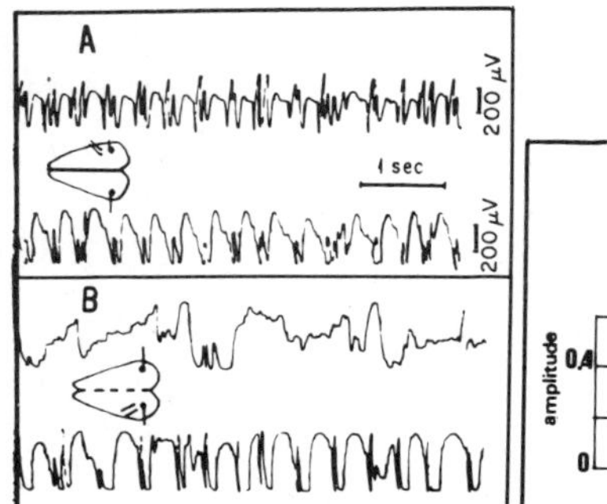
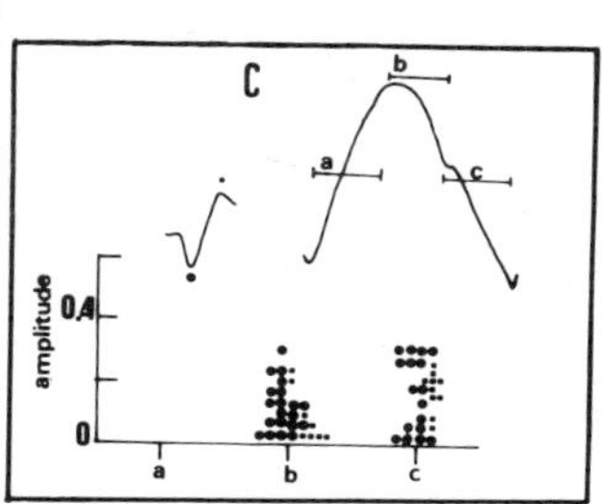

FIGURE 1-16. Self-sustained 3-per-second S–W discharges in the visual cortex evoked by direct epicortical stimulation A, before, and B, after, section of the callosal fibers. Acute experiment. Unanesthetized, artificially ventilated, paralyzed rabbit with bilateral lesion of lateral geniculate bodies. In C, attenuation (a) and lack of selective changes (b, c) of the positive (solid circle) and negative (solid square) phases of the primary potential on different parts of the wave of the S–W discharges. Ordinate indicates the amplitude in arbitrary units. Abscissa refers to the marked positions (a, b, c) of the wave on which the primary potential developed. (Compare with Figures 1-3 and 1-13.) The primary response was evoked by rectangular electrical stimuli applied through a concentric bipolar electrode in the white matter. Data based on the processing of averaged evoked potentials received in one acute experiment.

sides. We are referring, however, to the W–S discharge evolving from the SN–LR complex of the visual evoked response. Complexes of the same form (but probably of different origin) could be evoked in this preparation either by an increase in the dose of Metrazol injected intravenously or by the direct stimulation of the cortex with pulses of rectangular current. In both cases the S–W complexes emerged as a short fragment in the self-sustained electroconvulsive activity. Spike–wave discharges of this type are shown in Figure 1-16. Their bilateral synchrony is critically dependent on the integrity of the corpus callosum (Figure 1-16B) and they are easily distinguished from W–S discharges by applying a stimulus (for example, the stimulation of the cortical white matter) during various periods of the SN. Analysis demonstrated that almost no evoked response of the cortex could be observed in this case (Figure 1-16C). This convulsive discharge is probably identical with the one evoked in preparations of isolated cortex after the topical application of Metrazol or strychnine, or following some other procedure for creation of an epileptic focus.[4]

In some cases injuries in the mesodiencephalic area produced unstable EADs that appeared with a probability of .5 and less, or were quite regular, but weakly

---

[4] There are abundant data indicating that isolated islets of the neocortex can produce rhythmic activity. Perhaps this statement is disputable with regard to the regular alpha-pattern, but it is undoubtedly true for seizure rhythms, including forms similar to classical W–S discharges (Ingvar, 1955; Marcus & Watson, 1966). If they are not entirely new "isolation" phenomena, it might be useful to explain them on the basis of the *inhibitory*

expressed. In some cases an additional injection of Metrazol, a dose one-third that normally injected, evoked a stable bisynchronous rhythm of the W–S type. Figure 1-17 summarizes the effect of the entire series of experiments involving local subcortical destructions. Lesion locations are shown on only one side, although in most cases destruction was made simultaneously or subsequently also on the other side. The solid circles (the most effective lesions for W–S induction) are situated in areas whose electrical stimulation evokes behavioral and electrocortical arousal, accompanied by suppression of the EAD and the SEAD evoked by Metrazol injection.

Identical activity did not accompany the destruction of a number of other controlled points, and sometimes opposite effects were observed (suppression of

---

phasing theory. Such an explanation could throw light on the problem of the relations between W–S and S–W discharges.

It is well known that later (rebound) discharges are easy to evoke (if they are absent) or intensify by depolarizing a cell (by injuring it with a microelectrode, for instance). Such a cell immediately manifests rhythmic activity, albeit with some abnormal features.

In an oversimplified form it may be affirmed that the high frequency of firing is peculiar to the neurons in the epileptogenic focus created by an injuring agent (Ward, 1961). This means that exceedingly powerful background excitatory synaptic activity, included by Eccles (1965) as one of the pacemaker mechanisms, creates special conditions for the rhythmic discharges. The physiological intensity of this synaptic drive is further elevated by powerful and prolonged IPSPs acting to synchronize and thus equalize periods of the maximal excitability of the epileptic neurons.

It has been established by Matsumoto and Ajmone-Marsan (1964a, b) that during focal epileptic discharge neurons manifest an intense paroxysmal depolarizing shift. The level of the depolarization plateau of paroxysmal depolarization (PD) generally reaches 30 mV and over, and its duration is dozens of milliseconds. It may be preceded by slower depolarization, resembling ordinary EPSPs. The amplitude of impulses against a paroxysmal depolarization background varies depending on its size, and the impulses are often fully suppressed according to the mechanism of "Vvedensky inhibition" (cellular hyperdepolarization with the inactivation processes). This never happens with W–S-type discharges.

It would seem that in this case, too, the impulse activity of the cells activates inhibitory interneurons. As a result, paroxysmal depolarization is also followed by continuous waves of hyperpolarization (of a duration of 200–600 msec) with properties of typical IPSPs. In the elements, especially those on the periphery of the focus of epileptic activity, hyperpolarization waves emerge without preceding PD. Thus, an epileptogenic lesion facilitates the activity of a circuit that also meets the requirements for a W–S-rhythm pacemaker. But these focal discharges, even if identical in shape, are dissimilar with regard to their origins and properties. They reflect the activity of a subsequent stage of epileptization, when neuronal activity acquires features the elements of the normal adult cortex does not possess (Okujava, 1969; Prince, 1968a, b).

The S–W rhythm is determined by the same principle of recurrent inhibition circuits at the cortical level. But the presence of a hyperdepolarization effect, the increased sensitivity of the cell to synaptic activation, tends to produce a self-sustained convulsive rhythm in potentially any area of the brain, including isolated islets of the neuronal tissue and even tissue cultures. That is why I feel that it is useful to distinguish these S–W discharges from the W–S rhythm discussed in this book.

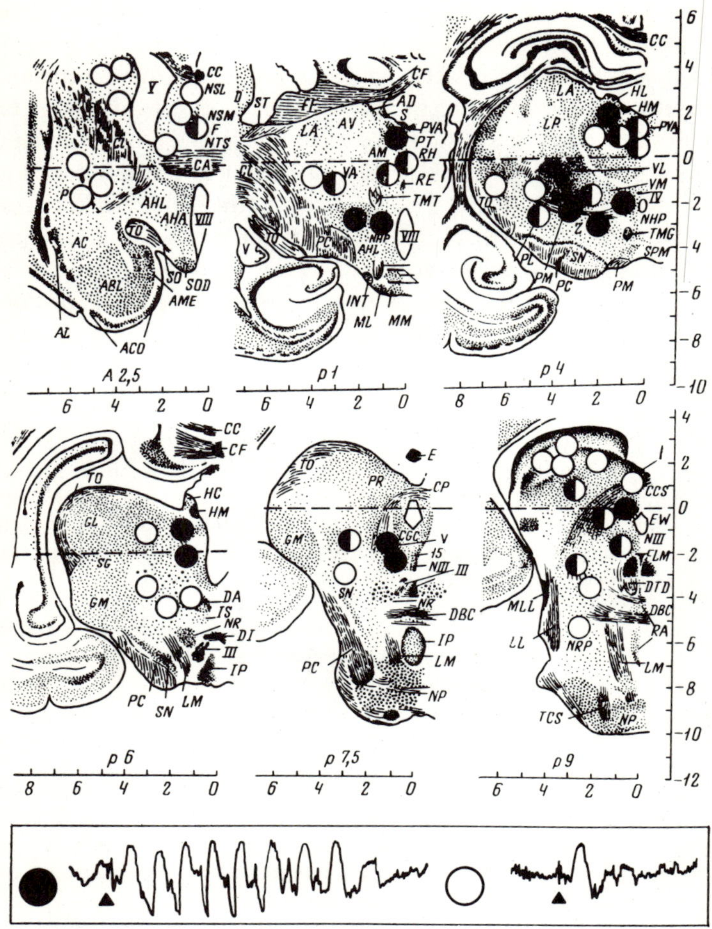

FIGURE 1-17. Summary data on the localization of destructions in the subcortical areas of the brain made on the basis of an analysis of the Nissl preparations. Brain sections after the stereotaxic atlas of Fifkova and Marsala (1967). Solid circles, sites leading to W–S activity after they were lesioned. Open circles, no EEG effect. Black-and-white circles, partial (threshold) or unstable effect. AC, nucleus centralis amygdalae; ACO, nucleus corticalis amygdalae; AD, nucleus antero-dorsalis; AHA, area hypothalamica anterior; AHL, area hypothalamica lateralis; AL, nucleus lateralis amygdalae; AM, nucleus anteromedialis thalami; APL, area preoptica lateralis; AV, nucleus antero-ventralis; CC, corpus callosum; CCS, comissura colliculi superioris; CF, comissura fornicis; CL, claustrum; CP, comissura posterior; DA, nucleus Darkschewitsch; DBC, decussatio brachium; E, epiphysis; EW, nucleus Edinger-Westphal; F, fornix; GL, corpus geniculatum laterale; GM, corpus geniculatum mediale; HL, nucleus habenulae lateralis; HM, nucleus habenulae medialis; IP, nucleus interpeduncularis; LA, nucleus lateralis anterior; LL, lemniscus lateralis; NRP, nucleus reticularis pontis; NSL (NSM), nucleus septalis lateralis (medialis); P, putamen.

synchronized activity and SN after such a lesion in the septum and orbitofrontal cortex). This indicates that epileptiform discharges emerged apparently as a result of lesions in structures involved in the control of cerebral rhythms, and that failure of this restraining apparatus leads to the release of the autonomous synchronizing thalamocortical specific inhibitory circuits. The idea of the irritative pacemaker in the site of the lesion seems improbable in these cases.

If such a subcortical pacemaker of the experimental W–S-type rhythm does exist, the most likely candidate is the specific thalamic nucleus, the lateral geniculate body. This is in effect a continuation of the theory of Eccles (1965) and Andersen and Andersson (1968) for W–S discharges developing from the sensory theta-rhythm. Although this conception was first formulated for the sigma rhythm, it is now the most attractive general theory for an explanation of the organization and metamorphosis of most cortical rhythms.

A microphysiological analysis of the activity of the projection cells of the lateral geniculate body (LGB) indicated (see Guselnicov & Supin, 1968 for a review) that the activity of these elements is identical with that of the ventro-basal complex (Andersen & Andersson, 1968; Eccles, 1965). During stimulation of the visual nerve or presentation of a light flash a microelectrode introduced into the LGB registers an initial negativity, accompanied by action potentials, followed by a long-lasting positive wave and subsequent negativity.

The intracellular analysis of this activity demonstrated that continuous positivity (P-wave) observed on extracellular records is formed by synchronous hyperpolarizing potentials (IPSPs), disrupting the initial depolarization. The latter was not always accompanied by action potentials, and this did not affect the duration of the IPSP or the rhythmical activity in a given cell. This suggests the possibility that postsynaptic inhibitory pathways in the thalamic specific nuclei as in the cortex are collateral and mutual.

According to Eccles' model of rhythmic activity (1965) the relay cells recovering from IPSPs would be in a state of hyperexcitability and display a tendency for a rebound depolarization. The rebound again reactivates the recurrent inhibitory mechanism and thus sets up a new cycle of inhibition and rebound discharges. Eccles (1965), however, does not exclude the excitatory synaptic action of special excitatory interneurons as a supplementary mechanism for the later (rebound) discharges on the thalamic level.

Taking into account that EAD and SEAD disappear after the destruction of the lateral geniculate body, one is tempted to assume that the visual relay cells may act as a pacemaker for the W–S rhythm in a manner similar to that postulated for the alpha activity. It seems very likely that the later discharges in cortical cells are at least partially controlled by a corticopetal volley from relay cells in which rebound discharges are well developed. According to this view further coordination of the synchronizing mechanisms at both levels is effected by the corticothalamic pathway. It terminates in particular on the inhibitory interneurons of the relay nuclei and exerts a hyperpolarizing action on their principal elements (Burke & Sefton, 1966a,b).

It appeared that cortical ablation eliminated intravenous Metrazol-induced W–S afterdischarges to a photic stimulus in the lateral geniculate. This may show that coordination of activities of both the neocortical and relay levels is important to W–S organization.

THE EFFECT OF HYPERSYNCHRONOUS CORTICAL ACTIVITY ON CONDITIONED REFLEXES

It was difficult to accept the idea that cortical phenomena, SN–LR, and sensory theta-rhythm should lead to a state resembling petit mal in a manner similar to that of the W–S discharges. For this reason we investigated characteristics of conditioned reflex elaboration against a background of experimental W–S. We felt that this would be a convincing and sensitive index of the slightest sign of "loss of consciousness."

This research was first conducted by Varga, Kuznetsova, and myself (1970a,b) on intact rats. A classical defensive reflex was conditioned. Photic stimuli, evoking sensory afterdischarge (SAD) in the visual cortex, were naturally used as the conditioning signal. A pair of electrodes was implanted, their isolated tips located under the skin of the nose, and stimulation via this means was used as the unconditioned signal.

In most animals rhythmical stimulation of the nose at about 40 Hz with rectangular current pulses (duration 0.5 msec, amplitude 15–20 V, and pulse series duration of 1–2 sec) evoked a washing reflex that continued some time following stimulation. In the event of more intense stimulation the washing reaction was replaced by a generalized locomotor–defensive pain reaction. Therefore, every test was begun by determining the threshold of the washing reaction, and when the threshold rose in the course of the experiment the intensity of stimulation was also increased.

Five light flashes with an interval of about 1 sec (flash energy was 0.3 joules) were used as the conditioning signal. The strobe was placed above the experimental chamber. The walls and floor of the chamber were made of mirrors and this ensured uniform illumination in any position the animal adopted relative to the light source. Reinforcement occurred simultaneously with the fourth flash and lasted, depending on the threshold of the washing reaction, from 1 to 2 sec. Not more than 20 combinations were presented per session and animals were given only one session a day.

The evoked potential to a light flash in the visual cortex of rats consists of the primary positive–negative or purely negative complex, maximum at 18–20 msec, and sometimes preceded by a low-amplitude negative oscillation. This is followed by the secondary "later" positivity with a maximum at 60 msec, and a slow negative wave (SN) with a maximum at 150–180 msec. The SN can end in a negative–positive or positive–negative–positive later response (LR). Usually the SN is preceded by a shorter additional negative oscillation with a peak latency on the order of 70–80 msec. Following a single light flash the SN–LR complex may repeat several times, as in rabbits, and form a characteristic series of waves or waves and spikes (SAD) (Figure 1-18A) (Kimura, 1962; Klingberg, Pickenhain, & Neumeister, 1967).

The first experiment showed that the sensory afterdischarge in rats generally appears in a state of quiet wakefulness; arousing or painful stimuli, unfamiliar conditions, and the like lead to its suppression. Small wonder, therefore, that when conditioned stimuli were presented with unconditioned ones SAD was suppressed and its first complex, SN–LR, was even extinguished. The conditioned reflex appeared after 4–15 trials (on an average, after 9 trials) and by trials 15–60 (on the average, by trial 30) was sufficiently strong. It was expressed in the animal by alertness, rearing, and the washing reaction.

In some cases the defensive components of the response predominated: The animal shook itself, pulled in its head, slowly retreated, made sudden jumps, fled to the corner of the box, or began to run wildly about the box, looking at the strobe. Immediately following presentation of the unconditioned signal, and in the course of establishing the reflex, the components of the sensory afterdischarge began to decrease and fragment; they finally disappeared completely (Figure 1-18B, C). The extinction of conditioned reflexes, on the other hand, was accompanied by the restoration of the SAD afterdischarge (Figure 1-18A).

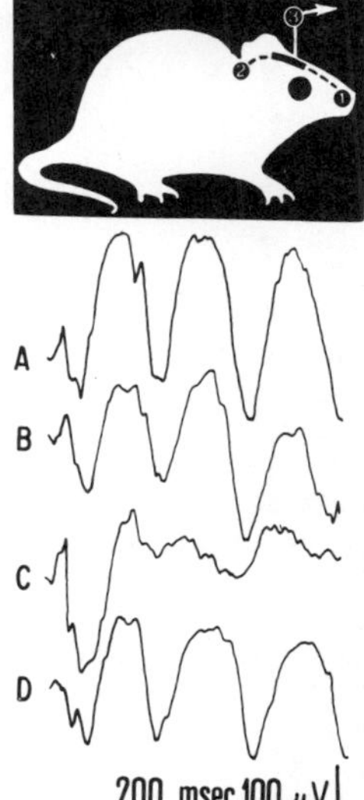

FIGURE 1-18. Changes in the sensory afterdischarge in the visual cortex during the classical defensive reflex in the rat. A. Background afteractivity to a flash. B. The beginning of conditioned reflex elaboration. C. The suppression of the afterdischarge in the period of stable reflexes. D. Rebound of afteractivity with the extinction of the reflex. The diagram shows chronically implanted (1) stimulating, (2) myographic, and (3) cortical electrodes.

A systematic analysis was made of these changes by counting the number of waves of the sensory afterdischarge during conditioning and extinction (Figure 1-19A, B).

Attention must be drawn to two relationships clearly expressed in the graphs. First, suppression of the SAD proceeds in parallel with an increase in the probability of the conditioned reflexes. When the SAD is initially not clearly expressed or when it is suppressed totally, the reflex is elaborated more rapidly. As the probability of manifestation of the conditioned reflex increases, the depression of the afterdischarges deepens. The degree of their later restoration is in direct relation to the degree that the conditioned response is extinguished. Second, it follows from the conclusions reached earlier that when a series of light flashes is used as a conditioning signal, the SAD to each sequential flash of light decreases as it approaches the moment of reinforcement, and maximum suppression is observed when the unconditioned current is applied.

Thus, the main result of this study was the providing of data on suppression of the SAD and its first component SN−LR during the establishment of classical defensive conditioned reflexes in rats. It was also found that the strength of the unconditioned electrocutaneous stimulation was of particular importance in suppressing the SAD. Therefore, additional series of experiments were performed involving the use of electrocutaneous reinforcement of different intensity.

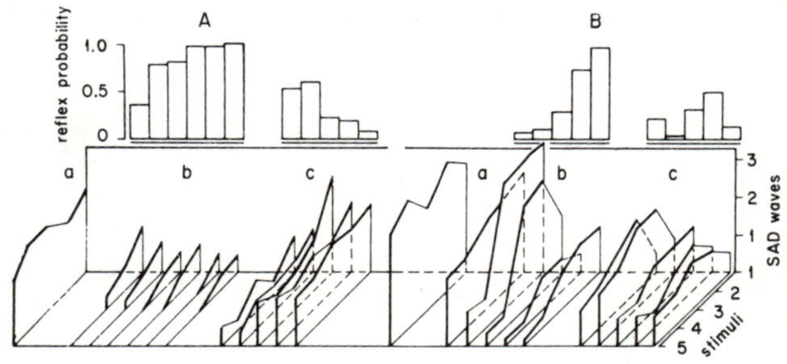

FIGURE 1-19. Dependence of the sensory afterdischarge dynamics upon the stage of classical conditioned defense (washing) reflex in the rat. Two normal rats (A, No. 12, and B, No. 39) having chronically implanted electrodes were used: a, sensory afterdischarge in response to a series of nonreinforced light stimuli; b, process of reinforcement during reflex elaboration; c, conditioned reflex extinction. Each plane in a–c reflects a mean number of waves (or wave—spikes) in the SAD to each flash (from a series of five flashes) comprising the conditioned stimulus during 20 trials with reinforcements or nonreinforcements. Note that as the period of reinforcement approaches, the afterdischarge becomes briefer. During electrical reinforcement, it is totally suppressed. For the same period (20 trials) reflex probability was calculated and plotted (in columns) above the corresponding plane. The more prominent the sensory afterdischarge, the smaller is the probability of the reflex. In rat No. 39 (B) more prominent and stable SAD is correlated with a delay in the stable conditioned-reflex formation.

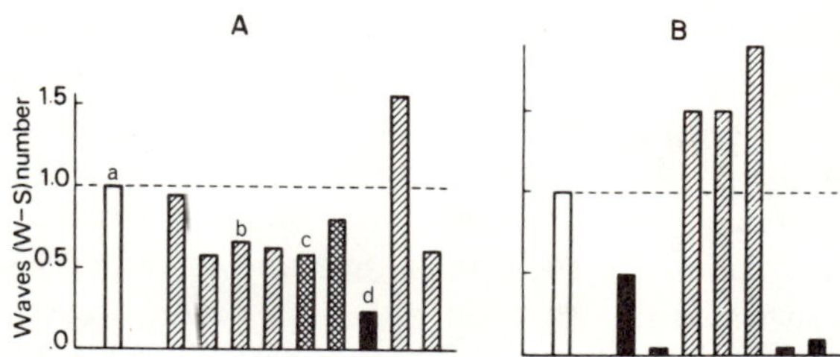

FIGURE 1-20. Changes in the duration of the SAD with changes in the physiological intensity of reinforcing stimuli. A, rat No. 45. B, rat No. 56. Ordinate, number of waves in afterdischarge in arbitrary units; a, before reinforcements; b, stimuli evoking one to two washing movements; c, reinforcement evoking more than two washing movements; d, stimulus strength evoking clear defensive or flight reactions.

It was found that the degree of suppression of the SAD during the establishment of defensive conditioned reflexes depends on the strength of the electrocutaneous reinforcement administered. On the whole, the SAD was much better expressed for less intense currents (Figure 1-20). The SAD is particularly facilitated when weak nonconditioned stimuli are used following a period of reinforcement with strong electrical stimulation. The exaltation of the SAD proceeds against the background of the animal's general tranquilization. Sometimes this is accompanied by light drowsiness, and the probability of the expression of conditioned reflexes decreases.

It thus seems that for successful conditioning electrocortical activity must be desynchronized. In other words, since the establishment of the defensive conditioned reflex takes place after suppression of synchronized activity, it is possible that the latter interferes with the process of conditioning. This is in itself a certain indirect indication that sensory afterdischarges, if they are strong and do not submit to desynchronization during the presentation of the unconditioned stimulus, make the establishment of conditioned reactions less probable. Indeed, in Figure 1-19B we see that the establishment of the conditioned reflex is greatly delayed in a rat with well-expressed sensory afterdischarges.

It must be admitted that even some time prior to these experiments data obtained by Livanov (1962) justified drawing the same conclusion. It was found that cessation of defensive reinforcement is accompanied by a synchronization of electrocortical activity. This blocked conditioned reflexes that had previously been elaborated but not subjected to extinction. Livanov (1962) refers also to the unpublished studies made by his associate Korolkova, who noted that the appearance of synchronization in the course of periodical extinction always coincided with the omission of the reflex, but restoration of the reflex coincided with the development of desynchronization. Every time a synchronized rhythm appeared in the cortex, all reflexes previously established in the stereotype were omitted. In the absence of synchronization these reflexes remained uninhibited.

At that time, however, Livanov was thrilled to observe the development of local and distant synchronization of the EEG in the theta band during the initial stages of learning. This other synchronous rhythm, which disrupted conditioning and contradicted his theory, was only briefly mentioned in the concluding section of the paper cited. It was not recognized at that time that there were two different rhythms. One was a stress theta-rhythm (hippocampal theta) whose appearance was always facilitated during the initial stages of conditioning. The other, a sensory theta-rhythm, was suppressed in this period, especially when the defensive conditioned reflex was elaborated. Correspondingly, it was facilitated during extinction of defensive conditioning when stress theta-rhythm was suppressed. These two rhythms are mutually exclusive.

It is natural to expect that conditioning will be more clearly suppressed when hypersynchronous rhythms of the EAD and SEAD type are developed. This assumption was studied in a special series of experiments (Varga, Kuznetsova, & Myslobodsky, 1971).

Figure 1-21, composed in a manner similar to Figure 1-17, shows the areas in which destructions were made in 32 rats and indicates their effects, using the symbols used in the earlier figure. Following destruction in the epithalamus or subthalamus, the typical evoked potential with afterdischarge of 1–3 waves evolved into an exalted afterdischarge (EAD). There were as many as 10 waves, or more accurately W–S complexes. In some cases this was accompanied by an increase of up to 300 msec in the duration of other waves in the afterdischarge, while in the background EEG W–S oscillations of the SEAD type were observed.

Elaboration of the conditioned reflex was begun 7–10 days following surgery. Figure 1-22 compares typical data from an intact rat and an experimental rat having W–S exalted afterdischarges resulting from bilateral coagulation of the habenular nuclei. In the intact rat the conditioned reflex was quickly established, and as the number of trials increased, there followed a reduction in the number of sensory afterdischarge waves. Virtually no afterdischarges were observed during the period of strong conditioned reflexes. In the experimental rat the afterdischarges were initially much more pronounced and they only decreased slightly during the time of electrocutaneous reinforcement. It will be seen from the figure that the conditioned reflex could not be established in 100 trials, and in most rats with a stable EAD it was impossible to establish conditioned reflexes even after 200 combinations.

In some rats with lesions in the area of the subthalamus and epithalamus the W–S EAD was less stable from the very beginning of learning, or it was normalized during the 10 days of trials. Accordingly, even though conditioned washing in these animals was elaborated, after a great many learning trials, the reflexes remained unstable. And here, too, omissions of the reflexes coincided with bursts of EAD in response to the conditioned signal (Figure 1-23B, a, b).

In the control group, which included rats with lesions in various loci that did not evoke paroxysmal reorganization of cortical rhythms, the elaboration of

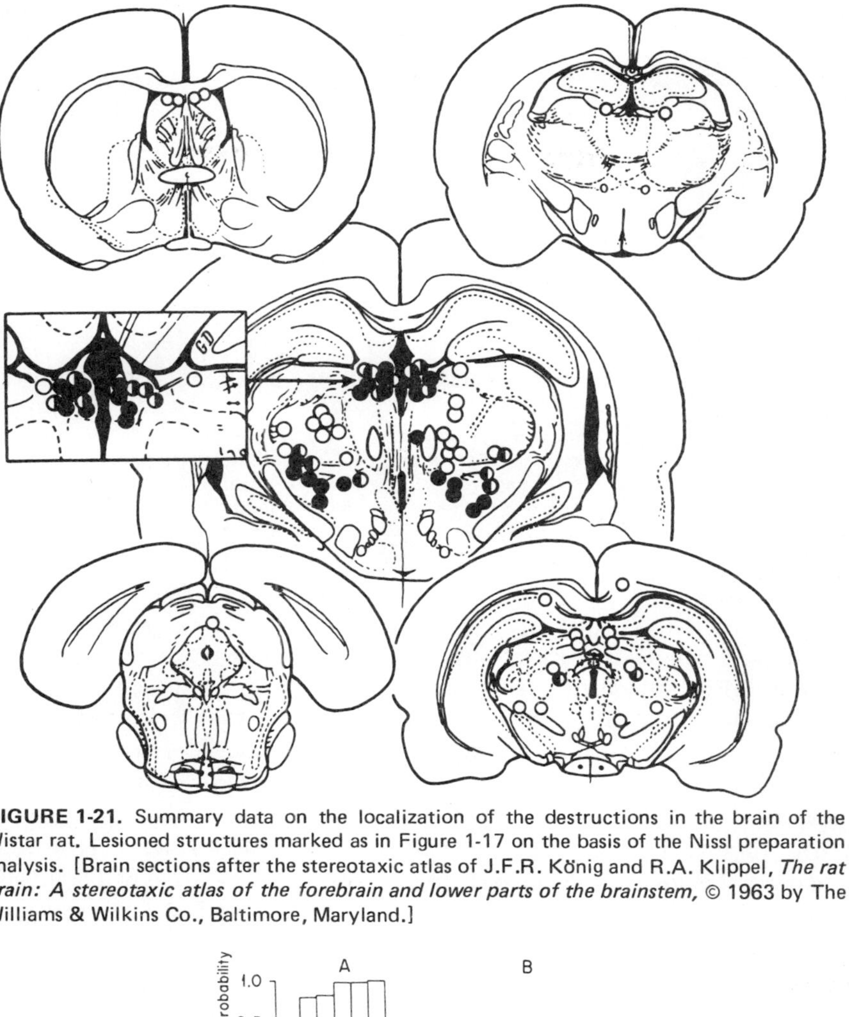

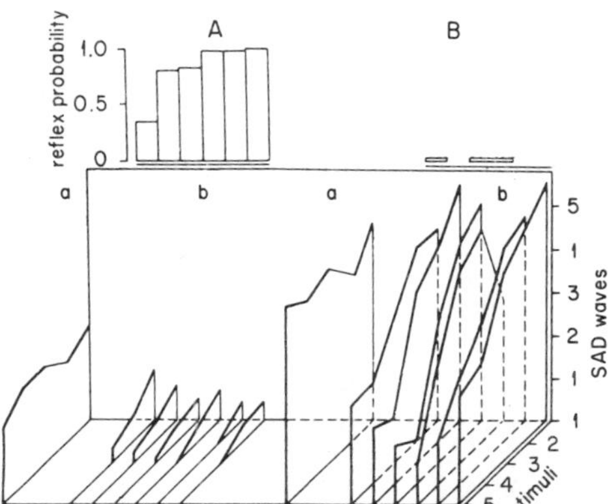

FIGURE 1-21. Summary data on the localization of the destructions in the brain of the Wistar rat. Lesioned structures marked as in Figure 1-17 on the basis of the Nissl preparation analysis. [Brain sections after the stereotaxic atlas of J.F.R. König and R.A. Klippel, *The rat brain: A stereotaxic atlas of the forebrain and lower parts of the brainstem,* © 1963 by The Williams & Wilkins Co., Baltimore, Maryland.]

FIGURE 1-22. Dynamics of conditioned reaction in A, normal rat and B, rat with bilateral lesion of habenular nuclei: a, background number of waves or wave–spikes in afteractivity to five light stimuli; b, the same after reinforcement. Upper columns reflect the probability of conditioned reflex. (See Figure 1-19 for explanations.) Note the absence of conditioned reflex correlated with prominent W–S afterdischarges.

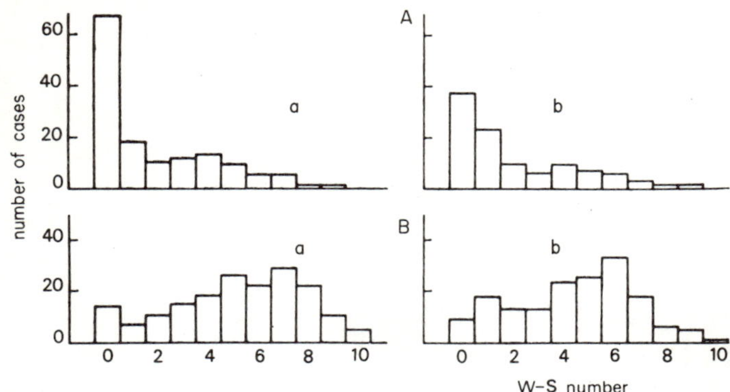

FIGURE 1-23. Histograms characterizing intensity of W–S afteractivity during A, appearance and B, omission of conditioned reflexes in rats with a, bilateral epithalamic and b, subthalamic lesions. In a, five light flashes were used as conditioning stimuli (CS); in b, flashes were paired with clicks. The ordinate shows the number of cases; the abscissa shows the number of waves in the EAD. In a, summary data were received from three rats; in b, data were received from four rats.

conditioned defensive reflexes to light took place at different times (from 4 to 70 trials). By the hundredth trial a firm conditioned reflex had been acquired by most animals. As stated previously, in most of these rats the afteractivity was of the ordinary SAD type. During elaboration of conditioned defensive reflexes these were suppressed and the general picture resembled that of the nonlesioned animals.

If it is true that the appearance of EAD interferes with learning, the formation of a reflex should not be disturbed by stimuli of a different modality that do not evoke a hypersynchronous EEG response. A series of experiments was performed to check this assumption. In four experimental, two control (lesioned but without EADs), and one intact rat, conditioned defensive reflexes were elaborated to a series of short auditory stimuli (clicks). Reflexes were established in all these animals relatively quickly—within 20 to 40 trials. Once strong conditioned reflexes were obtained, the clicks were presented in combination with light flashes.

In the intact rat and in one control rat this combination did not produce appreciable external inhibition, even when first presented. After further training the conditioned reaction grew stable. In one control rat the combined application of light flashes and clicks inhibited the previously established defensive reaction. However, following further presentation of the combined stimulus the conditioned reaction fully recovered. At the same time, the experimental rats displayed a large number of conditioned reaction omissions (Figure 1-23B, b).

Thus, it can be concluded that the inability to display a conditioned reaction is the result of the development of hypersynchronous activity of the W–S type.

The fact that the complete suppression of conditioned reflex activity did not take place in all experiments does not contradict this conclusion. In clinical practice, too, cases of incomplete loss of consciousness have been registered during petit mal (Lennox, 1960); and this has also been corroborated by special studies (Chatrian, Somasundaram, & Tassinari, 1968; Gibberd, 1966; Melnitchuk, 1971). In the experiment and in clinical studies this can be linked to qualitative and quantitative distinctions in the W–S discharges, which have so far been impossible to determine accurately. Indeed, when we made another behavioral test, the results were dissimilar to those described previously.[5]

The classical drinking reflex was elaborated in a manner similar to that used for the defensive reflex. The conditioning signal consisted of 10 photic stimuli with a frequency of 1–2 Hz. A drinking tube containing a 16% sucrose solution was presented with the fifth stimulus and was available for several seconds after the cessation of the conditioning signal. Rats were kept on a water-deprivation schedule and received liquid only during experimental sessions.

This conditioned reflex was elaborated in 15–30 trials, and no more than 40 trials were required to establish a very stable reflex. In the period of strong reflexes an additional behavior was conditioned: The rat had to run to a "drinking hole" (the tube was introduced through this hole) during the first five conditioned flashes and to drink the liquid without interruption the entire time it was available. Otherwise the nipple of the tube was withdrawn from the experimental cage. This required some 10–20 additional trials.

An analysis of the EEG and evoked potentials revealed that SAD changes in the process of learning passed through three main stages (Figure 1-24):

1. Brief fragments of SAD developed only to the photic stimuli coinciding with licking. (Reflex probability between .1 and .3.)
2. SAD began to appear to the first two nonreinforced flashes, was suppressed during the next two to three stimuli, and reappeared during most of the drinking period. (Reflex probability between .3 and .6.)
3. Constant SAD developed to every stimulus, especially to that coinciding with reinforcement. Owing to the slight decrease of SAD duration evoked by the fourth and fifth stimuli of the conditioned signal, the two-phase pattern of SAD dynamics seen in the preceding stage was preserved. (Reflex probability between .6 and 1.0.)

Thus, during the classical conditioned drinking reflex the SAD was a constant correlate of the stable conditioned reaction. But during extinction of the reflex, or during its failure, the SAD was usually suppressed. These data compel us to consider the possibility that in situations of defensive conditioning the SAD does

---

[5]This study was begun together with I. A. Kolomeitseva and continued with the help of Yu. K. Lapin, one of my students.

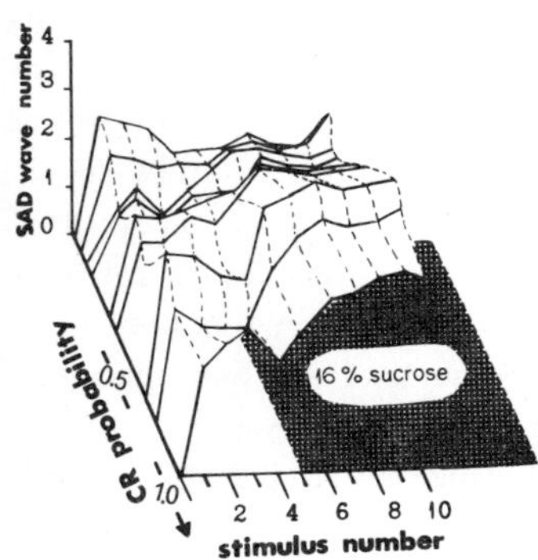

FIGURE 1-24. Three-dimensional graph reflecting interrelation of sensory afterdischarge development to each flash of a 10-stimuli conditioned signal and alimentary (drinking) classical reflex (CR) probability. The vertical axis indicates number of waves (or wave–spikes) in the afterdischarge. The horizontal axis shows the ordinal of the unconditioned stimulus number and the time of the reinforcement. On the CR probability axis is the conditioned reflex probability. The hatched area indicates the time of 16% sucrose presentation. Note the gradual increase of the sensory afterdischarge duration with the increase of the reflex probability. Each individual curve is derived from five trials.

not suppress the behavioral response by inhibition of the cortical mechanisms responsible for the processing of an incoming conditioning signal. Instead it may disrupt the normal functioning of the reward system. This disruption may be experienced by a rat as a false sensation of comfort and safety during SAD development, "misleading" the executive reticular mechanisms. This induces the rat to remain placid in the vicinity of painful stimuli.

At the same time, SAD dynamics during the drinking reflex demonstrate that this explanation can only be partly true at best. If one assumes that the SAD inhibits defensive conditioning by producing a drive-reduction state created by the synchronized EEG, the question then arises as to why the same SAD does not eliminate the drinking reflex. It could reduce drive in this case as well and signal that the body does not have any urgent requirements, such as for water.

To substantiate every point in this brief discussion would compel us to digress to the more general problem of reinforcement and its interrelation with petit mal epilepsy. The reader is referred to one of the concluding sections of this

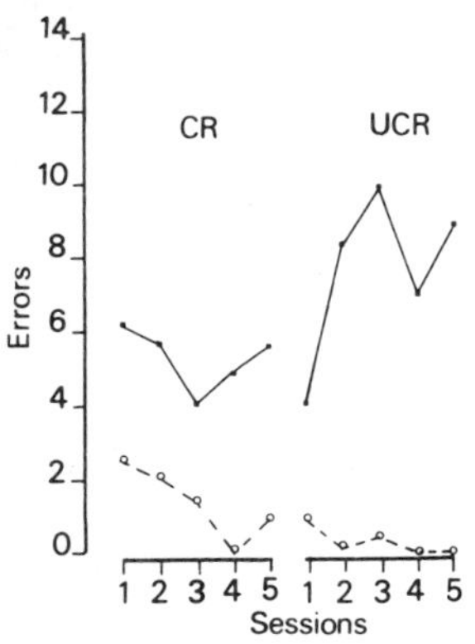

FIGURE 1-25. Disturbances of a stable alimentary (drinking) conditioned reflex after the intraperitoneal injection of small amounts (3–5 mg/kg) of Metrazol. CR (conditioned reflex) refers to omissions of the reflex during the presentation of the conditioning signal; UCR (unconditioned reflex), to disturbances of behavior during unconditioned stimulus presentation (short periods of drinking, omissions of unconditioned response). The ordinate indicates mean number of errors (omissions) or incorrect responses during conditioning stimulus and unconditioned stimulus presentation for a period of 20 trials (one session). The abscissa shows an ordinal number of sessions studied. Results are for a group of three Metrazol-pretreated (solid line) and control (saline-pretreated) animals (broken line). See text for further explanation.

book for a discussion of conditions where the SAD may interfere with drinking conditioning in the way demonstrated in Figure 1-20B. However, it is important to demonstrate here that the synchronization developed during drinking could suppress goal-directed behavior only when animals are pretreated with Metrazol.

Three rats with a strong drinking reflex were injected with small amounts of Metrazol (0.3–1.5 mg/kg) intraperitoneally. This is a subthreshold dose for W–S (EAD) development, but it stabilized the SAD. Five minutes later the rats were placed in the experimental cage for a regular session of 20 trials. Injections were made prior to conditioning every other day for 5 days (5 experimental sessions per day), and for every session SAD composition and reflex probability were evaluated. Three saline-injected rats served as a control.

Figure 1-25 summarizes the results of this series. It shows that the behavior acquired some new features. First, the probability of the conditioned reaction was lowered to about .7–.8. Saline injection also led to omission of the reflex, even though this reflex seemed to be very strong. At first glance this reflex derangement may be explained by external inhibition or by the orienting reflex, developing as a result of changes in the habitual situation. But omissions in the two groups may occur for different reasons. Indeed, several reflex omissions in saline-injected rats were correlated with a somewhat suppressed SAD, but this was never observed in the Metrazol-pretreated group. Thus the external inhibition hypothesis is not equally valid for the experimental rats and for the control group. The occurrence of a certain normalization of the reflex in saline-injected rats during the fifth session also supports this assumption.

Another feature of reflex derangement is that errors occurred during the presentation of the unconditioned stimulus. The unconditioned reaction in a thirsty rat is very strong and the rat drinks continuously when water is available. Metrazol-pretreated rats stopped licking every now and then. These episodes were counted as errors and plotted in the graph on Figure 1-25. It shows that such behavior was seen frequently (between 20% and 50% of the trails) and was not characteristic of the control animals.

Some Consequences of Embryonal Brain Injury

Up to 49.1% of all progradient cases of epilepsy (Kruglova & Rubinova, 1968), including "centrencephalic" forms, are ascribed to disturbances of prenatal development. However, it has been impossible either to prove experimentally that prenatal injury can lead to organization of inhibitory hypersynchrony of the W–S type or to enumerate the possible causes of the emergence of this inhibitory hypersynchrony. There has been even less progress in attempts to model genetic variants of petit mal. At the same time, it is only such models that ultimately will be able to test the many existing hypotheses on the nature of absences.

Recall that a lesion caused by the action of a damaging agent during the embryonal period of development may very closely resemble a mutation defect. An embryonal injury damages the same elements of the enzyme–chemical cycles that govern development processes, and these may also evince shortcomings caused by defects in the genetic code. In other words, a mutation is the result of a disturbance of ontogenesis brought about by insufficient or abnormal development of some fermentative systems. The same mechanism operates in embryopathy, except that in this case inactivation of the fermentative systems results from the direct action of a pathological agent, and not from defective genetic information. Such embryopathies, named *phenocopies* (Friesen, 1935), are apparently not hereditary, but are copies of genetic diseases, gene embryopathies (Svetlov & Korsakova, 1960).

By studying embryopathies, we are beginning to understand also the nature of the errors in genetic information leading to genuine epilepsy. Among the factors responsible for embryopathies, radiation injury is of special interest. It is recognized that X-irradiation is a potent epileptogenic factor (Geets, 1968), and it is a very convenient method of affecting embryonic development of the brain. Hence, the peculiarities of epileptization of the brain by prenatal injury will be considered on the basis of roentgenogenic embryopathies.

RADIOSENSITIVITY OF NERVOUS CENTERS IN ONTOGENESIS

In Western literature *radiosensitivity* refers to the degree to which cells and tissues are affected by the action of ionizing radiation. In the Russian literature this meaning is not considered sufficiently precise, and M. Livanov (1962) has proposed that a distinction be made between the concepts of *radioderangement* and radiosensitivity. The former is determined according to morphological criteria (let us say the degree and time of necrosis), whereas the latter is based on functional disorders. This definition could be reformulated in neuroanatomical or biochemical terms to avoid ambiguity, but a discussion here would serve no useful purpose. With respect to prenatal effects this subdivision has only theoretical importance; the concepts of radiosensitivity and radioderangement coincide here, and "functional" defects are generally a result of morphological injury.

An embryo's specific reaction to X-irradiation is determined by its age, since those elements developing most energetically at the moment of irradiation are the first to be destroyed. In other words, the sensitivity of tissues to X-irradiation is directly proportional to the intensity of the cell-division processes going on in the tissues and thus is inversely proportional to the degree of their differentiation. As early as 1906 this was formulated as a law relating the sensitivity of tissue in the fetus to the intensity of its metabolic processes (Bergonie & Tribandeau, 1964).

In embryogenesis the most radioresistant elements are neuroectodermal elements and medulloblasts, which are undifferentiated in the neuroblastic direction, i.e., the precursors of the neurons. They are not even injured by radiation at lethal doses. When they begin to transform into neuroblasts, the radiosensitivity of these cells increases dramatically and they become a target for penetrating radiation. Thus, it was established that in the course of development from the neuroepithelium to mature neurons, maximum sensitivity is displayed by postmythotic migrating neuroblasts (cell death is usually attributed to radiochemical damage to DNA) (Hicks, 1957, 1958). The threshold dose of the neuroectoderm (the minimum dose destroying the elements 2–8 hr after radiation) lies within the limits of 700 R. The postmythotic neuroblast perishes at a dose of 20–40 R, but the sensitivity of the young neuron decreases steeply again to 400–800 R. No structural damages are sustained by mature neurons, even from doses of 1000 R or more (Caveness, Carsten, Roizin, & Schade, 1968). Manina (1964) holds that mature neurons of adult animals structurally resist even enormous doses of ionizing radiation (up to 22,000 R) that exceed the dose causing mass destruction of neuroblasts by 500 times and that causing damage to nondifferentiated neurons by 200 times. It is astonishing that, in animals who perished with acute radiation sickness, the neurons of the central nervous system displayed no noticeable structural defect. Only a subsequent increase of the dose, which produces a most acute instantaneous form of radiation sickness, revealed that some neurons had sustained damage. However, in this case, too, the cortical elements were found to be in satisfactory condition.

It is clear that the nature of the pathogenic effect of radiation depends first and foremost on the period of antenatal development at which penetrating radiation is applied. In accordance with the traditions prevailing in embryopathology these effects are classified as *blastopathy, embryopathy,* and *fetopathy.* Strictly speaking, the last two are not phenocopies, for they are not really produced by a disturbance of the forming process but emerge as a result of the disease of the fetus caused by penetrating radiation (Piontkovsky, 1964).

Such fine distinctions may not be necessary to appraise the pathogenesis of radiation-induced disturbances of the brain structure. One of the important theoretical generalizations of the pathology of development is that of the relatively nonspecific action of harmful agents during the period of prenatal development. It has been established that the critical periods coincide for a vast group of harmful factors. A disease of the fetus may be a factor that to a certain extent reproduces the effects of radiation damage and reinforces and aggravates defects already caused by radiation.

In rats irradiation produces a general lesion of the central nervous system up to the tenth day of embryonal existence. This is the presumptive stage of development when there is as yet no histological differentiation of the neuroectoderm. During this period, X-irradiation leads to atrophic phenomena, owing to hydrocephaly and abnormalities of the ventricular system, or to coarse teratisms like anencephaly. The development of all other parts of the body proceeds satisfactorily (Hicks, 1957, 1958; Manina, 1964; Piontkovsky, 1964). Later, when tissue differentiation begins, the nature of the lesion changes fundamentally.

Because of their heterochronous development, the sensitivities of the individual formations do not coincide in time. The differentiation of the entire central nervous system can be described as a sequence of critical periods (Stockard, 1921), and the development of individual centers creates a spatial–temporal mosaic of changing vulnerabilities. This variation in the differentiation of brain structures is the reason embryonal injuries caused by radiation may possess traits of local "extirpations" (Hicks, 1958).

In rodents the maturing of the reticular formation, the basal ganglia, and a number of centers in the limbic system occurs in the middle of the embryogenic period. Hence, when rats are subjected to irradiation on the twelfth day of their antenatal life, lesions are mainly concentrated in the Ammon's horn, basal ganglia, and diencephalon. Edema, cytosis, and vacuolization of the nervous elements are found in the reticular formation of the oral pole of the brain stem and in the medulla. These phenomena progress and grow more noticeable with age (Alexandrovskaya, 1959, 1962; Artiuchina, 1958).

The lower layers of the cortex mature during the same period. Hence, rats subjected to irradiation on the twelfth and thirteenth day of embryogenesis, and rabbits on the fifteenth, evinced a thinning-out of the lower cortical layers (layers IV-V), a disturbance in the orientation of the pyramids, and various pathohistological changes (Alexandrovskaya, 1962; Chernishevskaya, 1962). The sensitivity of the subcortical structures to penetrating radiation also decreases with maturation. Although exposure of rats (Hicks & D'Amato, 1963) and rabbits (Ivanitsky, 1966) to X rays during late embryogenesis is responsible for a certain underdevelopment of the brain-stem centers, most defects are localized in the pallium. This is because the primary cells, which migrate from the periventricular area and form the external layers of the cortex, surface in several "waves" at the end of embryogenesis. Naturally, the effect of radiation during that period is to damage severely the outer layers of the cortex (Alexandrovskaya, 1959, 1962; Berry, Clendinnen, & Ears, 1963; Hicks & D'Amato, 1963). This effect results when a relatively small dose (10–40 R) is given, and when the dose is increased, lesions also occur in the lower layers (Hicks & D'Amato, 1963). Rabbits exposed to X rays on the twenty-third day of their embryonal life displayed a thinning-out of the upper cortical layers with coarse atrophic changes, centers of thinning, and an atypical orientation of cells and their dendrites (Chernishevskaya, 1962; Kruglikov, 1961). Changes in the lower layers seem comparatively insignificant.

RATE OF DEVELOPMENT AND NATURE OF LESION OF VISUAL CORTEX IN RABBITS X-IRRADIATED IN UTERO

Writings dealing with the rabbit's visual cortex frequently described only impressions. Behavioral maturation of antenatally irradiated rabbits and peculiar abnormalities of their behavior (Kruglikov, 1961; Myslobodsky, 1965) require more detailed morphophysiological study for the purpose of learning to what extent they should be attributed to nonspecific antenatal organic brain injury.

Geinisman and I (Geinisman & Myslobodsky, 1966; Myslobodsky, 1965) have compared the nature of cortical defects with the rate of development in two groups of prenatally X-irradiated rabbits. Radiation was carried out on the fifteenth or twenty-third day of pregnancy with the help of RUM-11 X ray apparatus. Working conditions were as follows: voltage, 190 kV; current intensity, 15 mA; filters, 1 mm Al + 0.5 mm Cu; dose capacity, 20 R/min; dose, 400 R.

It was known (Ivanitsky, 1955) that cortical cells in a normal rabbit's brain preserve their embryonal nature up to the twenty-third day of prenatal life. Their protoplasm stains poorly and the nuclei contain large amounts of chromatin. Tigroid emerges only at a definite stage of neuronal maturity, and is thus a unique indicator of the degree of maturity in the process of transformation from a neuroblast to a neuron. Initially the tigroid is found in the Cajal–Retzius cells, which are the first to mature. The first mature cells in layer V are found in newborn animals. By the sixth day of life mature cells predominate; all the cells of that layer mature by the tenth day. The cells of layer VI mature later, although some forms can be found in newborn animals. The bulk of the neurons on this layer mature by the eighth day; full differentiation of the elements is only completed by the thirteenth day. The cells of the upper layers begin to differentiate later and also complete their development later. The first to mature are the pyramids of layer III, followed by the cells of layers II and IV. In the granule cells, tigroid emerges during the second week of life. By the end of the second week all the cortical cells have definitive structure, and no further substantial changes are observed in the structure of the neurons.

In a pilot study, Geinisman and Myslobodsky (1966) found that in irradiated animals most of the cortical cells were mature by the end of the first week of life. For a more quantitative description of this effect, the differentiation of neurons, as observed in Nissl preparations and with the histochemical reaction for RNA, was subdivided according to Ivanitsky (1955) into three main stages:

1. *First-Stage Maturity.* The cell has a roundish form. The nucleus is round and diffusely colored. There may be several small nuclei of equal size. The cytoplasm is poorly developed: A thin rim of cytoplasm envelops the nucleus or concentrates on one side. The cytoplasm color is lighter than that of the nucleus.
2. *Second-Stage Maturity.* The cell body becomes oval or pear-shaped. The nucleus grows lighter, and its coloring loses its diffusive nature. The cytoplasm acquires a more intensive coloring than the nucleus. Its structure is homogenous.
3. *Third-Stage Maturity.* This is the stage in which the transformation of the neuroblast into a mature nerve cell takes place. The neurons acquire a definite form: Granule cells are irregular or star shaped, pyramidal cells take the typical triangular form. The cell nucleus is light-colored and one large nucleus clearly stands out against the background. The amount of cytoplasm increases noticeably and surrounds the nucleus on all sides. Granules of the tigroid appear in the cytoplasm.

Thirty X-irradiated rabbits were used for morphological study. The brains of the control and irradiated animals were studied on the eighth and twelfth days of their postnatal life. For each age period the brains were sectioned at 10 μ or at 7 μ, and processed with the help of the histochemical reaction for RNA.

Within the limits of the cortical layer in both hemispheres the number of cells was counted in a space of 600 μ^2. The number of cells of different degress of maturity was expressed as a percentage of the total number of neurons. The data thus obtained were analyzed statistically, and the results are presented in Tables 2-1 and 2-2.

On the eighth day of life (Table 2-1) most of the cells in the visual cortex in normal rabbits fit the second maturity stage, and the number of cells in the third stage is negligible. An exception are the cells of layer V, which, as mentioned previously, mature earlier than other cortical neurons. The cortical elements of 8-day-old animals in both X-irradiated groups are much more differentiated than in the control animals. In the irradiated animals most cells in all cortical layers correspond to the third maturity stage.

On the twelfth day of life (Table 2-2) the degree of cell differentiation between control and experimental animals is negligible. By that age most cells in

TABLE 2-1. Degree of Cortical Maturation of Control and X-Irradiated Eight-Day-Old Rabbits (in Percentage of Cells at Each Maturity Stage) [a]

Cortical layer	Control			X-Irradiated on fifteenth day in utero			X-Irradiated on twenty-third day in utero		
	1	2	3	1	2	3	1	2	3
II	10.7	85.9	3.4	12.3	47.3	40.4	5.5	19.3	75.2
	9–14	83–99	2–4	9–15	43–51	36–44	3–7	16–22	71–78
III	2.4	97.6	–	–	29.4	70.6	7.4	21.3	71.3
	1–3	97–99			25–33	67–75	5–9	18–24	67–75
IV	8.7	91.3	–	6.0	56.1	37.9	3.6	46.4	50.0
	7–12	88–93		4–8	52–60	34–42	3–6	42–50	46–54
V	–	55.1	44.9	–	20.2	79.8	–	26.6	73.4
		51–59	41–49		17–23	77–83		23–31	69–77
VI	3.1	95.8	1.1	2.1	45.4	52.5	2.1	32.4	65.5
	2–4	94–97	0–2	1–3	41–49	48–56	1–3	28–36	62–70
II–IV	7.3	91.6	1.1	6.1	44.3	49.6	5.5	29.0	65.5
	5–9	90–94	0–2	4–8	40–48	46–54	3–7	25–33	62–70
V–VI	1.6	75.4	23.0	1.1	32.8	66.1	1.1	29.5	69.4
	1–3	71–78	20–27	0–2	29–37	62–70	0–2	26–34	65–73

[a] 95% confidence interval is marked under each mean.

TABLE 2-2. Degree of Cortical Maturation in Control and X-Irradiated Twelve-Day-Old Rabbits (in Percentage of Cells at Each Maturity Stage)[a]

Cortical layer	Control		X-Irradiated
	2	3	3
II	16.3 13–19	83.7 81–87	100
III	2.4 1–3	97.6 96–99	100
IV	11.0 9–14	89.0 86–91	100
V	3.0 2–4	97.0 96–98	100
VI	1.3 0–2	98.7 97–100	100
II–IV	9.9 8–13	90.1 87–92	100
V–VI	2.1 1–3	97.9 96–99	100

[a] 95% confidence interval is marked below each mean.

all the cortical layers of the control animals have attained a definitive type. However, elements that fit the second maturity stage are found in the control animals, whereas none are found in the experimental animals.

Initial perusal of the preparations led us to believe that thinning out of the cortex was occurring in the experimental animals. To check this observation and to obtain more precise information on the locus of the radiation lesion we made a quantitative analysis of changes in the size of the transverse section of the visual cortex.

The results, given in Table 2-3, show a thinning out of the visual cortex in both groups of experimental animals on the eighth and twelfth days of life. However, the predominant site of the lesion was different in each group. In animals subjected to X-irradiation on the fifteenth day of embryogenesis, thinning was observed in the upper as well as the lower floors of the cortex, although the deep layers (V–VI) were more affected. This thinning was clearly seen on the twelfth day of life. In rabbits irradiated on the twenty-third day of embryonal development, thinning occurred predominantly in the upper layers (I–IV).

TABLE 2-3. Mean Thickness of Visual Cortex Layers in Control and X-Irradiated Rabbits (in μ ± Standard Error)

Cortical layers	Control	X-Irradiated on fifteenth day in utero	X-Irradiated on twenty-third day in utero
		8 days after birth	
I	123.40* ± 2.29*	110.41 ± 2.17	108.13 ± 1.83
II–IV	341.57* ± 7.89*	281.37* ± 6.06	263.35 ± 6.17
V–VI	432.28* ± 7.09	392.73* ± 9.37	426.33 ± 7.54
		12 days after birth	
I	164.59* ± 1.74*	125.08* ± 2.60	141.24 ± 2.29
II–IV	409.03* ± 5.37*	323.11 ± 5.20	324.25 ± 7.80
V–VI	520.63* ± 6.86	420.63* ± 5.23	539.76 ± 11.54

*$p < .001$.

The selective lesioning of the cortex by prenatal X-irradiation at various periods of embryogenesis indicates the high radiosensitivity of these layers at the moment of exposure to X rays. This, however, does not explain the damage suffered by the molecular layer in animals subjected to irradiation in late embryogenesis, or the damage to the upper layer of the cortex in rabbits X-irradiated in the middle of their embryonal development (Table 2-3). The periods of maximum radiosensitivity of the elements in the indicated cortical layers do not coincide with the time of the X-irradiation. The most probable explanation is that these changes are secondary. Indeed, the molecular layer is made up of terminal branches of the upper dendrites, mainly of pyramidal and spindle-shaped cells of the lower cortical layers. Dendritic branches and glial elements make up the main mass of layer I; it contains a relatively small number of cells (Cajal, 1955). Fibers of axonal origin are also among the main elements of the molecular layer. They form a dense net, interweaving with the dendrite plexus. It should be noted that some of the axonal fibers forming layer I ascend from the subcortical brain formations (Cajal, 1955; Lorente de No, 1943). This explains the great vulnerability of layer I, which always bears some marks of lesions initially affecting other layers of the cortex or subcortical formations.

When animals are subjected to radiation during late embryogenesis and injury is inflicted on cortical layers II–IV, the molecular layer is also affected. This apparently occurs because a large number of dendrites from the affected nerve cells do not participate in the formation of layer I. The effect on this layer from X-irradiation during midembryogenesis is probably due to lesions of the lower cortical layers and the nonspecific formations of the brain stem (Ivanitsky, 1966; Piontkovsky, 1964). Recall that the dendrites from the cells of layers VI and V and axons ascending from the nonspecific formations of the brain stem branch out in the molecular layer (Cajal, 1955; Lorente de No, 1943). Therefore, it is likely that irradiation decreases the degree of participation of these elements in the formation of layer I. A similar mechanism appears to be responsible for thinning in layers II–IV of the visual cortex in rabbits irradiated on the fifteenth day of embryogenesis.

It follows that the lesion of layer I should be more clearly expressed in animals X-irradiated on the fifteenth day of embryogenesis, since the lower cortical layers, as well as the nonspecific system of the brain stem, are affected. This is indeed the case; it is clearly manifested on the twelfth day of life (Table 2-3).

It was also shown that in 12-day-old animals, irradiated on the fifteenth day of embryonal development, the number of cells in the upper cortical layers was virtually unaffected, but in the lower cortical layers about 13% of the neurons perished. In contrast, in rabbits irradiated at the end of embryogenesis the number of nerve cells in the lower floor did not differ substantially from that in control animals; in the upper floor a diminution of up to 26% was registered. The decrease in the transverse section of the lower cortex floor in animals irradiated on the fifteenth day is probably due to both the destruction of cell elements and the fiber structure. The destruction of 13% of the cell elements cannot explain the drastic thinning out of lower cortical layers in these animals (Table 2-3).

It may be concluded that in rabbits irradiated on the fifteenth day of embryonal development lesions first localize in the lower cortex layer. There is also indirect evidence suggesting derangement in the subcortical brain structure. In rabbits irradiated on the twenty-third day of embryogenesis, the primary radiation lesion is limited to the upper cortical layers.

In addition to causing the obvious local structural disturbance of the cortex and subcortical centers, exposure to X rays accelerates the development of nervous tissue. This accelerated development was shown by Purpura and Shofer (1968) in the ontogenesis of Purkinje cells in the cerebellum of kittens. The interrelation of the two effects, destruction and acceleration, is of special interest.

An analysis of Table 2-1 shows that the localization of the maximum defect coincides with the maximum acceleration of cell development. This is particularly clear in rabbits irradiated on the fifteenth day, when the maximum number of cells in the third stage of maturity is located in the lower layers. In rabbits irradiated on the twenty-third day, however, the number of mature cells sharply increases in the upper layers. Since the development of the lower cortical layers anticipates the development of the upper, the acceleration effect is less noticeable from irradiation in late embryogenesis. Thus, conditions for accelerated development of nerve cells are created in the locus of the lesion for reasons as yet difficult to determine.

From the teleological viewpoint this reaction perhaps appears to sustain the life of the organism by hastening the exit of cells from their critical period, but at the same time it may have catastrophic consequences. Local acceleration lends the structure certain specific traits differing from those with which it normally develops. The result is a decay of the genetic program for the development and organization of intracentral and intercentral circuits. The further development of this new system is random and it is practically impossible to predict the result of the regraduation of intercentral relations, nor is it likely that such predictions will be made in the foreseeable future. Yet these effects may be helpful when analysis is made of the consequences of prenatal injuries to the human brain, especially of problems related to the lateralization of an epileptic focus, which I shall touch upon in a subsequent section. It is also useful to bear these facts in mind when an analysis is made of the effects of the acceleration of development, for precocious maturation may be accompanied by the development of an epileptiform syndrome (Elian, 1970).

SOME ELECTROPHYSIOLOGICAL CORRELATES OF PRENATAL BRAIN INJURY

X-irradiation is able to damage and even destroy entire areas of the brain or some of its structures. Naturally, a more or less localized lesion can be inflicted only if relatively small doses are applied.

It is therefore not surprising that in studying radiation-induced disorders of the central nervous system researchers soon discovered that its stable pathological changes are sometimes unique models for analysis of inborn brain diseases, laws of embryogenesis, rates of development, and aging (Hicks, 1958, Piontkovsky, 1964). The complexity of this approach is self-evident. It can be successful only if there is accurate information on the time of fecundation and the embryogenesis of the various brain structures. This condition cannot as yet be fully satisfied. Experimental embryology is today, as 40 years ago when the extirpation possibilities of prenatal radiation trauma were first realized, "in the embryonal stage of development [Hicks, 1958]." Even so, radiation techniques have the potential for local destruction of individual cortical layers; they have been used to analyze the nature and rates of development of primary and secondary responses in the visual cortex (Myslobodsky, 1964) and the cerebellum in kittens (Purpura & Shofer, 1968). Also, sensory afterdischarges and rhythmical responses to light have been examined in rats (Klingberg *et al.*, 1967).

In 1964 Piontkovsky advocated using radiation-induced embryonal injuries for modeling inborn endocrinal, cardiovascular, nervous, and psychic diseases. In the last group attention was focused on oligophreny, because disturbances of the intellect are frequently concomitants of embryonal injuries; the sad experience of Hiroshima and Nagasaki demonstrated that penetrating radiation produces such injury. Also neurodynamics, clinical data, and some peculiarities of the EEG revealed specific similarities between oligophreny and experimental postirradiation pathology (Airapetianz, 1966; Ivanitsky, 1966; Kruglikov, 1961).

On the other hand, it was found that animals who have sustained a prenatal injury of the brain and cerebellum also display epileptiform fits. In Long-Evans rats irradiated on the second day of their postnatal life with a dose of 500 R (total), a convulsive fit could be evoked 3 days earlier than in control specimens. Throughout their 2-month observation, the seizure threshold remained lowered, although the total duration of fits was shorter than in intact rats (Vernandakis & Timiras, 1963). In 50% of rats irradiated with 100 R on the fourteenth day of their embryonal life, complete tonic clonic seizures appeared 2 days earlier than in control animals (at 16 days after birth) and were distinguished by greater acuteness (Vernandakis, Curry, Maletta, Irving, & Timiras, 1966).

Miller (1962) irradiated mice from the first to the thirtieth (γ-irradiation with cobalt-60, dose 0.14 rad) or between the twenty-third and the thirtieth day after birth (total dose 1.5–2 rad). Even with such an insignificant dose, irradiation decreased the latent period and increased the acuteness and frequency of audiogenic seizures.

In an experiment made by Cooke, Brown, and Krise (1964) Wistar rats were irradiated with a dose of 2 R during the first 10 days of their embryonal life (γ-irradiation with cobalt-60, total dose 20 R). The irradiated offspring had lower thresholds for audiogenic seizures.

Werboff, Den Broeder, Havlena, and Sikov (1961) irradiated Sprague-Dawley rats, considered resistant to audiogenic seizures, on the fifth, tenth, fifteenth, or twentieth day of embryogenesis with doses of 25, 50, or 100 R. Lowering of the audiogenic seizure threshold was only observed in animals irradiated on the tenth or twentieth day of embryogenesis (examination at the age of 4 months). Irradiation on the fifth or fifteenth day, however, resulted in a noticeable increase in resistance to epileptic reaction. According to Sikov's data (quoted by Kimeldorf & Hunt, 1965), irradiation of rats on the fifteenth day with a higher dose (185 R) led to a significant increase in the frequency of spontaneous seizures and to the development of photomyoclonic reactions and audiogenic myoclonus. When the rats were irradiated with a dose of 50 R, convulsive seizures were absent; and no convulsive seizures were observed following irradiation with 20 and 100 R on the tenth day of embryonal life. Epileptiform reactions were more intense in males.

In rabbits irradiated with 400 R during the period of organogenesis frequent episodes of arrest reactions and rotating motions resembling running fits of rats were observed (Kruglikov, 1961). Slow waves, bursts of high-amplitude spindles, spikes, and other forms of paroxysmal activity were also observed (Berry *et al.,* 1963; Ivanitsky, 1966; Kruglikov, 1961; Piontkovsky, 1964). These phenomena were considered an indication of the stable shift of the equilibrium in corticoreticular relations, with a lowering of the intensity of ascending effects typical of the "adynamic variety" of oligophreny (Ivanitsky, 1966).

Naturally these data could also be interpreted as an indication of a radioembryological epileptiform syndrome, aggravating oligophreny. An organic lesion not only leads to an intellectual defect but also promotes the development of an epileptic process. This assumption could be tested because it had already become clear that the postradiation epileptiform syndrome was a reality.

Kolomeitzeva and I (1969) made studies of brain reactivity in Chinchilla rabbits irradiated on the fifteenth and twenty-third days of embryogenesis.[1] Rabbits irradiated in midembryogenesis were on the whole more restrained, and unresponsive at 5 to 6 months of age. They proved more submissive than normal rabbits during fixation, and their orienting reflex was extinguished more rapidly. Even though some did not differ noticeably from control animals, a simple measure of motor activity indicated that they were one-third less active than normals. Some specimens displayed a completely paroxysmal advent of freezing, which was not observed in normal animals at all.

The second group of control animals, subjected to radiation in the twenty-third day of prenatal life, did not display even traces of nonreactivity. It was interesting to note that these rabbits sometimes displayed atypical aggressiveness. They reacted with a characteristic thumping behavior when they were approached or handled. Fixation evoked ferocious resistance, and the orienting reflex was remarkably stable and difficult to extinguish.

Of particular interest were the observed paroxysms of behavioral inhibition displayed by rabbits irradiated on the fifteenth day. This phenomenon was also described by other writers who defined it as *catalepsy* (Piontkovsky, 1964). Similar effects observed in conditioned reflex experiments were always interpreted in terms of Pavlovian physiology, as a result of disturbances in force, mobility, irradiation, concentration, and balance of nervous processes. Understandably, if a similar phenomenon is encountered in humans, at least an EEG is made to determine whether the disturbance of neurodynamics is the consequence of periodic bursts of hypersynchronous waves and whether these accompany disturbances of consciousness affecting the behavioral performance.

---

[1]Conditions of X-irradiation were practically the same as described above: filtered (0.5 mm Cu + 1.0 mm Al) X rays (dose 300 R; dose capacity 15 R/min, voltage on the tube 190 kV, current intensity 15 mA, focal distance 50 cm).

Such an analysis was made in this case. It revealed two facts. First, the entire group of rabbits irradiated during the period of organogenesis displayed a typical, synchronized EEG and a corresponding evoked response to light. The secondary SN–LR complex was particularly intense, and this was reflected in the appearance of episodic EAD in the visual and central areas of the cortex.

In later analysis of EEGs six animals displaying particularly clear symptoms of "freezing" were selected from those irradiated on the fifteenth day, and more intense indications of hypersynchronization were revealed. They were displayed by the emergence of diffuse and bilaterally synchronous bursts of waves in the theta–delta range and complexes of paroxysmal 2.5–4-per-second W–S discharges that coincided with the arrest of ongoing behavior.[2]

The forms of hypersynchronous waves produced by flicker in a mature prenatally irradiated rabbit resemble those that normally emerge only after Metrazol poisoning or injury to the oral pole of the brain stem (see Chapter 3, Figure 3-5). They are distinguished by greater generalization and lower frequency. Since the frequency of the rhythm is mainly determined by the duration of the IPSP, it follows that injury in midembryogenesis somehow increases the effectiveness of postsynaptic inhibition. This conclusion was tested in a study of the extracellular unit activity in the visual cortex of prenatally irradiated animals.

Recall that the reacting elements can be divided into four groups in accordance with their response to light (see Table 2-4). Of the normal animals, 16.9% responded only with short latency spikes (type I). In 19.3% there was an initial inhibitory period followed by a later ("rebound") discharge (type II). In 29.9%, cells reacted with initial and later discharges, separated by an inhibitory pause (type III). Type IV resembled type III, but the inhibitory pause was interrupted by action potentials with a probability on the order of .5. These cells were counted separately because they were so numerous—33.9%.

In animals irradiated on the fifteenth day, there was a statistically significant increase in the number of units responding as type II (49.4%) and a 20% increase in the duration of their inhibitory phases. There was also a corresponding decrease in the number of cells reacting according to types I and IV. Irradiation on the twenty-third day of embryogenesis was used as a second control, and only affected the incidence of type III cells, which increased to 43.1%.

Changes registered in the visual evoked potentials in the two groups of

----

[2] These episodes of hypersynchronization were not immediately apparent and their discovery was somewhat accidental. Once, after a number of unsuccessful attempts to produce a W–S rhythm in irradiated rabbits, it was decided to interrupt the experiment. When the researchers returned 2 hr later, they found many records with clearly marked complexes of spontaneous bursts of W–S-type activity. This experiment made it clear that a lowering of the arousal level to produce W–S discharges is not just a theoretical prerequisite, especially when the animals studied are restrained.

TABLE 2-4. Mean Number of Visual Units Having Different Response Patterns in Control and X-Irradiated Rabbits (in Percentages)

Response pattern	Control	X-Irradiated on fifteenth day in utero	X-Irradiated on twenty-third day in utero
I	16.9	3.6**	12.1
II	19.3	49.4**	17.2
III	29.9	31.4	43.1
IV	33.9	15.6*	27.6

* $p < .05.$

** $p < .001.$

irradiated animals are essentially opposite. SN–LR was facilitated in rabbits irradiated on the fifteenth day and suppressed in those irradiated on the twenty-third day. This leads one to suspect that the effect is mediated by the reorganization of interneural circuits, at least on the cortical level. Cells that respond to light with initial inhibition show that the inhibitory synaptic activities are addressed not only to those cells activating the given interneuron, but in a varying degree to all cells on which the collaterals of the inhibitory axon terminate. And these are elements of the second type. If an embryonal injury leads to an increase in elements responding in this manner, it is only natural to assume an increase in the number of collaterals of the inhibitory axons and, correspondingly, an increase in the probability of mutual inhibition. However, this effect may also be linked with other factors, such as an increase in sensitivity to inhibitory transmitter. At this stage it is preferable to speak of an increase in the effectiveness of the inhibitory synaptic action, without conjecturing about its mechanism.

An important point is that in addition to the growth of the probability of mutual inhibition, there is also a noticeable increase in IPSP intensity. This can be seen indirectly from extracellular recordings in the duration of the inhibition pause, its stability, and (with certain provisos) the probability of later discharges. Table 2-4 shows that the number of elements reacting with only an initial discharge is negligible in rabbits irradiated in midembryogenesis; the number of cells responding with a reaction of the fourth type is reduced by one-half. This indicates the regularity and high amplitude of IPSPs in these elements, and indirectly also characterizes the activity of the entire population. Up to 55.4% of the cells react to light with repeated cycles of inhibition–discharge activity, sometimes three to five times. Normally this is observed in 14.5% of cells, and it is entirely absent in rabbits irradiated on the twenty-third day.

Another point worth considering is that cells in X-irradiated animals fail to settle in definite cortical layers according to cell type. In the normal brain such topography can be seen from accurate vertical penetration of the cortex by a microelectrode. One may divide all cells into two major groups—active cells that fire during one of the phases of the primary reaction, and passive cells that react with initial inhibition and a later response. It will be noticed that these groups concentrate in different cortical layers. Active cells are concentrated in the midcortex at a level of 1.2 mm and in the lower layers at a level of 1.7–2 mm. Passive cells, however, are found primarily in the lower layers of the cortex. Within the heterogenous active group those elements that respond exclusively with a primary reaction have a nearly constant distribution along the vertical. This subgroup of active cells is found already at a level of .6 mm from the cortical surface and is most frequently encountered in its center. Virtually no such units are found below a level of 2.0 mm.

As was mentioned previously, the active cells are not a homogenous group. They are classified as a group because they are apparently the first to respond to an afferent signal. The passive cells become involved in the reaction because they are located in the field of action of the same inhibitory interneurons. A comparison of the latent periods of active cell discharges, however, shows that they differ. These cells were therefore subdivided according to the nature of their reaction and its correlation with the short latency or primary response. Accordingly, they can be divided into three groups:

1. Cells firing during the period corresponding to the positive phase of the primary response.
2. Elements firing predominantly during the following positivity of the primary reaction (latent period on the order of 40–60 msec).
3. Cells responding with equal probability during the first and second positive waves of the primary response.

The distributions of these cells vary across the different levels of the cortex. Cells of the first group are found from .6 mm and are most concentrated at a depth of about 1.1–1.2 mm. The cells of the second and third groups are found mainly in the middle and lower cortical layers. It is likely that their reactions are in some way linked with the specific anatomic organization of the net. This assumption applies, first and foremost, to the cells in the first group. These short latency elements, located in the midcortex, may be the pyramids of layers III–IV. Cells of the third group found at this level may be related to them.

It is much more complicated to imagine the role of the cells of the second group. Although they do not begin to discharge until 40–50 msec after the stimulus, they react with the longest high-frequency group discharges. Some of the cells of this group fire as many as 5–11 action potentials during the high-frequency group discharge, which is accepted as a characteristic of interneurons. However, it seems unlikely that these are inhibitory interneurons, because they cease discharging against the background of the SN and renew activity during the development of the LR. Their later discharges are more intensive than cells of other types. It is therefore more likely that these cells form part of the recurrent activating circuit. Such cells were discovered in the motor cortex (Humphrey, 1968; Takahashi, Kubota, & Uno, 1967), but it would be premature to explain the activity of the elements of the visual cortex on the basis of ephemeral analogies or indirect evidence.

In view of these data it is logical to expect that animals X-irradiated on the fifteenth day of embryogeny having lesioned lower cortical layers would show a diminution in the number of cells reacting with primary inhibition. On the other hand, changes in the number of these cells are not to be expected in animals X-irradiated on the twenty-third day of intrauterine life with a lesion predominantly located in the upper cortical layers. The most probable targets for this lesion are active primary responding cells of the upper and the middle layers. However, as described previously and in Table 2-4, the experimental results did not conform to expectation.

Perhaps the data would be in agreement with the theoretical prognosis if it were possible to lesion selectively upper or lower cortical layers in mature animals. But in this case the lesion was inflicted in a period affording wide opportunities for reorganization of neural contacts, and in the process of recovery a new circuit could be composed with different, mostly abnormal, properties. This is reflected partly in the lack of order in the distribution of active and passive units across the visual cortex.

The question remains why in both groups the very cells whose elimination was expected were predominant. Compensatory increase in the lesioned population does not seem to be the likely explanation. The pattern of a cell's reaction is a property of the circuit to which it belongs and not of the cell itself. Thus something happened to the circuits, and above all to the inhibitory circuits, that led to changes in the reaction pattern of a large population of cortical cells and stimulated an increase in the number of units having a definite type of reaction.

Hence, another hypothesis might be suggested. It is believed that there was derangement of mechanisms controlling the activity of the inhibitory circuits, which resulted in facilitation of inhibitory synaptic action in one case (irradiation of the fifteenth day of embryogeny), and diminution of that action in the other (irradiation on the twenty-third day). Disinhibitory influences may be considered a result of the activity of special inhibitory cells that block inhibitory interneurons (inhibition of inhibition) postsynaptically, or moderate activities of the interneuron presynaptically.

The central assumption is that the executive mechanism for this control system operates by way of fibers ascending from structures of the limbic–reticular complex. Indeed, such a suspicion would arise from some direct (see earlier) and my own indirect data, which indicate derangement of the reticular formation in animals irradiated on the fifteenth day of embryogeny, and the release of its function in animals irradiated on the twenty-third day.

One of the most widespread and instructive techniques for studying inhibitory mechanisms of the cortex is to determine the threshold and other parameters of the electroconvulsive afterdischarge. (See Table 2-5.) True, this may be rather variable in rabbits (Straw & Mitchell, 1966), and it is more difficult to determine the time when the convulsive rhythm is completed than in cats. However, the variability of the characteristic is mainly due to experimental faults, such as damage to and drying of the cortex, hemorrhages, disturbance of hemodynamics, and fluctuations in depth of narcosis. The test may be considered acceptable only if its duration is decreased and the experimental conditions are standardized.

Electroconvulsive afterdischarge was produced in unanesthetized paralyzed rabbits, artificially ventilated and fixed in a stereotaxic device. The surgery in this case was usually conducted under ether narcosis. From 1.5 to 2 hr following inhalation of ether vapors a special plate made of organic glass with pressed-in stimulating and recording electrodes was placed on the visual cortex. Stimulation was begun at 4–5 V, and every 5 min the voltage was increased by 1–2 V until the first symptoms of convulsive activity were registered. The threshold was determined three more times with an interval of 5–7 min between tests. The stimulation frequency was 20 Hz; the duration of the pulse 1 msec; the duration of the rhythmic series 6 sec. Table 2-5 shows that in the offspring of rabbits irradiated on the fifteenth day of pregnancy the duration of the seizure afterdischarge was minimal, but its threshold did not differ from that of normals.

TABLE 2-5. Parameters of Electroconvulsive Afterdischarges in Control and X-Irradiated Rabbits (Mean ± Standard Error)

Parameters	Control	X-Irradiated on fifteenth day in utero	X-Irradiated on twenty-third day in utero
EAD threshold (mg/kg)	7.49 ± 0.41	3.09 ± 0.37*	6.06 ± 0.73
Photomyoclonic response threshold (mg/kg)	10.76 ± 0.46	5.15 ± 0.51**	10.00 ± 0.83
Seizure afterdischarge threshold (V)	11.30 ± 0.56	10.41 ± 0.62	8.30 ± 0.34*
Seizure afterdischarge duration (sec)	57.30 ± 13.10	47.60 ± 14.50	151.11 ± 41.13**

*$p < .001$.

**$p < .05$.

Contrariwise, in rabbits irradiated in late embryogenesis it was significantly lower, and its duration was three times that in normals.

I believe that the results of this experiment indicate higher convulsive activity thresholds in animals in which we have observed indubitable symptoms of an epileptization of the brain. A number of experiments established that tonic clonic forms of convulsive activity of the cortex are based on a progressive decrease of hyperpolarization waves, an increase in the duration of depolarization waves, and their temporary summation with Vvedensky inhibition phenomena, i.e., cellular hyperdepolarization with inactivation processes (Matsumoto & Ajmone-Marsan, 1964b; Okujava, 1969). Thus, the electroconvulsive afterdischarge is based on a derangement of postsynaptic inhibition and excessive depolarization of some low-threshold cells. Correspondingly, the extent of malfunction of the inhibitory apparatus of the cortex relates to the amount that the convulsive threshold is lowered. In any case, irradiation at the end of embryonal development leads to a noticeable disruption of synchronized forms of epileptic activity. In some rabbits there is a steep decline in the secondary SN–LR complex, a higher frequency of impulse activity, and an increase in the number of cells discharging with unstable silent period, IPSP (43%). The enumerated data are an adequate index of the weakness of postsynaptic inhibition in that group of animals and explain the probable cause for the rapid hyperdepolarization of the cortex during its surface stimulation.

Determination of the photoconvulsive and photomyoclonic thresholds was made in unanesthetized rabbits held in a special device with a headrest and ear-holder. Following the injection of Novocaine into the ear root and the intravenous injection of 50 units/kg of heparin into the lateral vein of the rabbit's ear, a 2.5–5% solution of Metrazol was injected with a velocity of less than 5 mg/kg per min. The dose of Metrazol administered ensured that the EAD would be evoked in not less than 5 out of 10 presentations of light stimuli. Then injection was continued until the photomyoclonic reaction appeared. Two experiments were made with every animal at an interval of 2–3 days.

In a normal rabbit the photoconvulsive reaction (EAD) appears at a dose of 7.49 ± 0.46 mg/kg. In rabbits irradiated in midembryogeny electrocortical activity was quite synchronized by overreactive postsynaptic inhibition and rebound discharges. These rabbits required 50% less of the drug for provocation of the EAD and photomyoclonus. At the same time thresholds were not altered in animals irradiated in late stages of embryogenesis (Table 2-5).

EX JUVANTIBUS APPROACH TO WAVE–SPIKE
DISCHARGE IDENTIFICATION

In cases of disease with unclear symptomatology it is possible to diagnose the illness by simply varying the type of medication. Such a *diagnosis ex juvantibus* is valid where very specific drugs acting on a narrow range of pathophysiological mechanisms are used. Actually researchers are very often in a position of diagnosing ex juvantibus since any diagnosis is more or less a hypothesis to be tested by the outcome of medication.

This approach can be used to study experimental W–S discharges, since successful antiepileptic medication depends upon the type of the seizure pattern. For example, trimethadione is of great value against petit mal, but is of no use in the treatment of grand mal or psychomotor epilepsy. On the other hand, Luminal (phenobarbital) has some value in petit mal treatment, but is a drug of choice against grand mal seizures. Another drug, diphenylhydantoin sodium, is of great value in the treatment of grand mal but is contraindicated in petit mal.

These three agents, representing the three important classes of anticonvulsant diones, barbiturates, and hydantoins were used in the following study. A group of 12 rabbits X-irradiated on the fifteenth day of embryogeny were selected for frequent EEG and behavioral abnormalities that could be considered as models of a petit mal fit. In all rabbits background EEGs and visual evoked potentials were repeatedly recorded, and the number of waves or W–S complexes in the SAD or the EAD was taken as a pretreatment measure of abnormal EEG reactivity. Rabbits were divided into three treatment groups. The maximum daily therapeutic dose of the drugs used in clinics (about 60 mg/kg for trimethadione and about 10 mg/kg for Luminal and diphenylhydantoin sodium) was injected intraperitoneally twice a day (8 AM and 8 PM) for 10 days. On the eleventh day EEGs and evoked potentials were recorded and the state of afteractivity in the visual cortex was inspected.

In only the trimethadione-treated group was hypersynchronous W–S afteractivity eliminated, although this group had shown the most constant and clear W–S activity before treatment. In the other groups W–S afteractivity remained unchanged after medication.

After an interval of 3 days, all rabbits previously treated with Luminal and diphenylhydantoin sodium were treated with trimethadione for another 10-day period. And again the result was unequivocal: Only the first component of the W–S afteractivity, the SN, remained, and usually it was reduced.

A similar study was conducted in eight rabbits bilaterally lesioned in the central gray matter and habenular nuclei. In all these animals W–S afteractivity was sometimes more prominent than in X-irradiated animals. To avoid interference with possible spontaneous EEG normalization, treatment was begun 2 days after the implanting of electrodes and lesioning of brain tissue and was continued for only 5 days. The effects of trimethadione and diphenylhydantoin sodium given in the same doses as described previously were compared in this series. Four rabbits were treated in each group. The results presented in Figure 2-1 show that only trimethadione was effective in suppressing W–S complexes.

The important effect of the trimethadione in both the X-irradiated and the lesioned animals was that it also improved behavior. Strict behavioral tests were

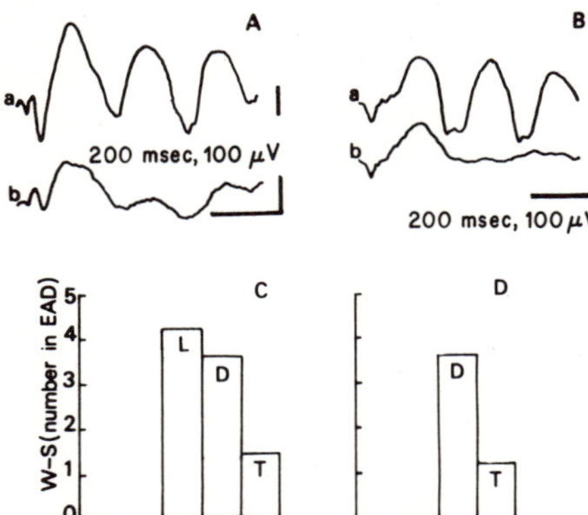

FIGURE 2-1. Effects of Luminal (L), diphenylhydantoin (D), and trimethadione (T) on W—S afteractivity in X-irradiated and lesioned rabbits. A, B. Averaged visual evoked potentials show individual results in A, X-irradiated and B, lesioned rabbits after trimethadione treatment: a, before treatment; b, after treatment. Average of 15 responses to a single light flash. Semirestrained rabbits with chronically implanted electrodes. The graphs show the group result of the treatment in (C) irradiated and (D) lesioned animals. The ordinate indicates the number of waves or W—S in the afterdischarge. Each group consisted of four animals.

not conducted in these studies, but ongoing behavior of the animals was always inspected and behavioral reactions to external signals were recorded. Recovered trimethadione-treated rabbits were distinctly more animated. They reacted with a strong orienting reaction to external stimuli and displayed locomotor exploratory activity, which had previously been minimal.

In this respect it is interesting to mention that the areactivity, periods of immobility, and the learning deficits of X-irradiated animals were attributed to progressive inborn pathology of the brain (Piontkovsky, 1964). There is no doubt that the acutely lesioned immature rabbits were as seriously affected, yet there was distinct electroclinical improvement in both cases. Thus behavioral derangement was a function of the selective lesion in certain brain structures. This in turn led to the EEG abnormalities that determined the periodicity and duration of the specific behavioral disorder.

This study, too, shows that the experimental W—S and SAD, or its first component, the secondary SN—LR complex, may be used as a sensitive instrument for the selection of new drugs with anticonvulsant properties. Support of this assumption came from an independent study of Shearer, Flemming, Bigler, and Wilson (1974) conducted in albino rats. Three anticonvulsants, Tridione (trimethadione), depakine (dipropylacetate), and Dilantin (diphenylhydantoin sodium) were tested for their effect on photically evoked SAD. It was found that all these anticonvulsants suppressed the SAD, although Tridione and depakine had greater effects. Data on the effect of trimethadione on W–S discharges and EADs in X-irradiated and lesioned rabbits are in good agreement with the research of Shearer *et al.* (1974) in normal rats. Although our studies failed to demonstrate any suppressive effect of diphenylhydantoin sodium, this could be because we used less than half the dose of Shearer *et al.*

3 Sensory Activation of
Wave–Spike Discharges

In this chapter the study of experimental W–S discharges will be continued in the field of photogenic epilepsy. Supersensitivity to flickering light develops when W–S discharges appear in the EEG. This phenomenon was stressed when peculiarities of some of the models of W–S were described (Guerrero-Figueroa *et al.*, 1963a, b; Morrell & Baker, 1961; Stevens *et al.*, 1964). It can also be observed in patients with petit mal epilepsy. Thus, there is the attractive possibility of finding a new dimension of similarity between the experimental W–S and that appearing in petit mal patients. It was also hoped that the application of traditional methods for studying photogenic epilepsy (such as investigation of recovery cycles) would help to clarify some mechanisms of W–S activity in general.

It is natural to question whether it is possible to activate an electroclinical photogenic seizure of the petit mal type in normal animals. If it is not possible, then perhaps those processes can be revealed that stabilize the reactivity of the normal brain, since it may be their derangement that leads to W–S development.

CAN PHOTOGENIC SEIZURES
BE EVOKED IN NORMAL RABBITS?

It was not possible to evoke a hypersynchronization of electrical activity resembling W–S discharges with ordinary rhythmical light stimulation either in the course of flicker or in its aftereffect. How does natural stimulation by light differ from electrical stimulation of the brain, which invariably evokes epileptiform disturbances of brain activity? Is it only that the discharges evoked by electrical stimulation are more synchronous? Apparently this is true for the epileptiform discharges of grand mal, but this can hardly be the main reason for the ineffectiveness of flicker in provoking a W–S-type rhythm. The latter does not require such a massive participation of cortical neurons, as was noted during study of cellular activity following Metrazol poisoning and during analysis of the impulse activity of the visual cortex in irradiated animals. The number of reacting neurons in irradiated rabbits is practically the same as in normals; the differences involve only the mode of reaction. Apparently, one should look for some stabilizing mechanisms that prevent change in the mode of reaction in normal cells during flicker.

Flickering-light stimulation at a frequency of about 10 Hz appears to grow brighter. If light of subthreshold or threshold intensity is used, the human subject sees episodic or correspondingly regular flashes at that frequency. This phenomenon is known in psychophysics as the *brightness enhancement* or *Bartley effect*. Bartley (1959) obtained the effect at a frequency of 8–10 Hz but noted that it can also be observed over a wider range of pulsations—from 2 to 20 per second. Lange (1954) also considers that maximum sensitivity to flicker emerges at a frequency of about 9 Hz, although he found that the first appearances of flicker (the stimulus was of a subthreshold intensity) were noted by the subject at 3.6 Hz and continued up to 14 Hz, disappearing at higher frequencies.

Thus, brightness enhancement is noticed at frequencies found to be epileptogenic. It is very likely that fluctuations in the excitability of cortical circuits occur with a frequency close to that evoking the brightness-enhancement effect. Coincidence of the external flicker frequency with the endogenous one leads to a considerable resonant increase in the excitability of the system. This is why Bartley (1959) and, later, other researchers advanced the theory that the brightness-enhancement effect is somehow related to processes similar to those of the alpha rhythm.

In a rabbit, stimulation with flicker at a frequency close to the basic electrocortical rhythm evokes a gradual augmenting and then a decreasing of the amplitude of the rhythmic evoked potential (potentials of driving). The dynamics of "waxing and waning" are usually associated with the rhythmic response to electrical stimulation of the specific and nonspecific nuclei of the thalamus, i.e., the augmenting and recruiting response. It will be referred to here as the *sensory augmenting response*. With reference to its shape, it is tempting to assume that in accord with Bartley's theory, intensification in the brightness of flicker coincides with the maximum of the evoked spindle, i.e., with the waxing phase. In this regard, the waxing phase of the sensory augmenting response may be viewed as the electrophysiological correlate of the Bartley effect, or as a correlate of the maximal sensitivity of the sensory system.

According to signal detection theory (Pollack, 1961), when the sensitivity of the detector is high the system is less stable and responds with a high false-alarm rate. Alternatively, if the critical response level of the detector is set high, the system should be very stable but proportionally less sensitive and may consequently fail to report many of the signals actually presented. It may be assumed that such terms as *high sensitivity, low stability,* and *high excitability* applied to the neural circuit or sensory system indicate a higher risk for epileptic response. Thus stability of the detector system is of no less adaptive value than its sensitivity. That is why a highly sensitive system should be less stable. It therefore seems that a compromise for the optimal stable and sensitive detector could be found if the sensory system could be only periodically sensitive for a limited amount of time. Specifically, a prediction for the sensory augmenting response was that there is a decrease in the stability of cortical cells synchronized by light pulsations (waxing). Then in the waning phase some mechanisms must operate that interfere with the high cortical excitability and divert cortical elements from their dangerous proximity to epileptic reactions. According to this assumption, extending the period of high-amplitude reactions, or delaying the waning phase of sensory augmenting, should enable us to register a burst of self-sustained hypersynchronous discharges of the type described in Chapter 2. However, to conduct such an experiment requires studying not only the composition of the rhythmic response but also the mechanisms regulating its amplitude.

Let me begin this section with a description of the visual evoked potentials (VEPs) to paired photic stimuli, since it is obvious that the nature of rhythmic reactions is derived from the cortical excitability cycle. If the VEP to the first of two stimuli is represented by all its secondary components, including the SN–LR complex, then the shape of the primary potential to the second stimulus varies with the interval between them. It appears to be immediately dependent upon the portion and parameters of the SN against which it develops. This sort of interference has already been demonstrated to verify the nature of the SN of the W–S complex (Figures 1-3 and 1-13).

The primary response to a conditioning stimulus is suppressed against the background of the following positivity of the primary reaction or at the very beginning of the SN. A similar picture is observed 200–250 msec later when the SN is completed. In both cases the testing primary response has a characteristic shape, which is due to the predominance of its negative phase. However, a stimulus presented at the top of the SN (150–170 msec), when it is just beginning to decrease, evokes an abrupt facilitation of the primary response. It exceeds that preceding by two to three times (Figure 3-1).

Similar, although somewhat weaker, interrelations are seen when stimuli are

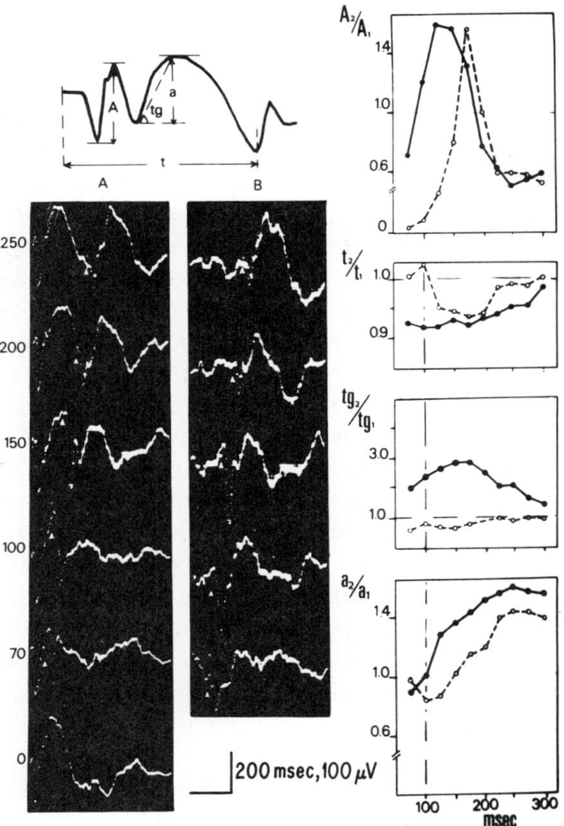

FIGURE 3-1. Visual evoked potentials to double photic stimuli in normal waking semire-strained rabbit. The second stimulus presentation is marked by an arrow; the first stimulus presentation coincides with the start of the analysis. Column B contains differential tracings corresponding to each averaged evoked potential in column A. The graphs show the recovery curves of different characteristics of visual evoked potentials in normal rabbits (solid line) and in rabbits having lesions in the central gray matter (broken line). A_2/A_1, recovery of the amplitude of primary potentials; t_2/t_1, recovery of the SN duration (or the LR latency); tg_2/tg_1, recovery of the SN steepness; a_2/a_1, SN amplitude recovery curves. Ordinate indicates the ratios described. Abscissa shows intervals between stimuli. Vertical interrupted line at 100 msec indicates the critical delay time when the presentation of the test flash only changes the characteristics of the potential to the first flash but does not evoke a clear potential (for lesioned animals only).

presented during different portions of the SN of the sensory theta-rhythm or of the SAD. Thus the dynamics of the primary potential to a second stimulus shows excitability changes taking place with the frequency of sensory theta-rhythm or SAD, and not a true recovery or restoration of cortical responsive-ness. This facilitated potential differs in more than just amplitude from the primary reaction to the conditioning stimulus. Its duration reaches 24.1 ± 0.6 msec when the duration of the positive phase of the primary response to light is 6.1 ± 0.4 msec. The time to the maximum of the positive wave generally exceeds 50 msec (51.3 ± 0.9 msec); the time to the summit of the positive phase of the primary response is 24.0 ± 0.5 msec. These characteristics are identical to those of the waxing potential of the sensory augmenting response, evoked by intermittent light with an interstimulus interval of 150–170 msec. This facilitation will be labeled as the *augmented potential (A-potential).*

The impression is often created that the testing primary response develops on the descending phase of the A-potential. When Nembutal is injected to suppress the SN, the A-potential is also suppressed and the VEP to a second stimulus acquires the appearance of a monotonous restoration cycle (Myslobodsky, 1966). The same type of restoration is also observed during suppression of the SN and sensory theta-rhythm by tetanization of the mesencephalic reticular formation or when spontaneous stress theta-rhythm (hippocampal theta) develops.

However, the presence of the SN is not the only requisite condition for this unique modulation of the afferent volley. After injection of benactyzine or atropine, the SN sometimes intensifies, but the restoration curves of the primary response acquire a rather monotonous appearance (similar to that following the injection of Nembutal), which stems from the elimination of the exaltation phase.

Note that both atropine and benactyzine suppress the LR. On the other hand, Nivalin, chlorpromazine hydrochloride, and Metrazol intensify the LR and facilitate the exaltation phase of the restoration cycle (Myslobodsky, 1966, 1973). It seems likely that the A-potential is activated by the same mechanism that underlies the LR. Thus, the A-potential forming the waxing phase of the light-induced augmenting response results from the heightened excitability of the cortex, which occurs close to the end of the SN and just before the LR.

But this does not explain why the A-potentials are waxing and subsequently waning. We must examine the dynamics of the SN–LR complex to a second stimulus to explain this phenomenon. A testing stimulus presented on the rising SN slope evokes a small primary potential; when delayed by about 70–80 msec it is rarely followed by a pronounced SN. The latter may sometimes be seen with the aid of averaging techniques on a differential curve (Figure 3-1). A distinct SN appears only with the first signs of A-potential development, and it reaches its maximum with the maximal manifestation of the A-potential. In this period augmentation of the SN is accompanied by augmentation of the LR and sometimes initiates a burst of several new SN–LR complexes of the SAD to a test stimulus.

It was mentioned previously that the amplitude of the A-potential is a function of the development of the SN–LR complex. It facilitates the response to a test stimulus presented with a delay of 150–170 msec, and this creates the background for a more powerful A-potential to the next stimulus. This has immediate implications for the waxing phase of the sensory augmenting response; the waning phase has as yet no explanation.

The intensification of the SN is often associated with an increase in the amplitude of the primary response, if the A-potential can be considered such. The A-potential evokes a more powerful discharge of cortical cells, which accordingly produce a more intense and synchronous inhibition. However, during the period when the A-potential was replaced by a low-amplitude primary response (delay of the test stimulus 200 msec or more), the SN amplitude and the steepness of its rising slope remained facilitated (Figure 3-1).

On the graphs in Figure 3-1, the decrease in duration and time to maximum of the SN of the test potential is due to increased steepness of the SN. In consecutive repetitions of these experiments we found a stable decrease in these parameters of the SN to a test stimulus by not less than 5–10%. Interestingly, the maximal decrease of SN duration with LR facilitation coincided with the maximal amplitude of the A-potential, and at larger interstimulus intervals its duration began to return to its initial level.

Since we had already concluded that the SN is a reflection of an IPSP in the depths of the cortex, it seemed logical to believe its decrease represented a lowering of inhibitory synaptic action. At the same time, this idea was contradicted by the increase in the LR amplitude, the organization of the SAD to the test stimulus, and the increase in the amplitude and steepness of the SN itself. I will discuss the nature of this phenomenon later. Now it is important to demonstrate how the SN duration decrease influences the response to a third stimulus, should one be presented following the same delay of 150 msec. Since the duration of the SN to the second stimulus is less and its front is steeper, the third stimulus does not register against the same SN portion as does the preceding stimulus. During a gradual shift of the SN summit, every new stimulus of the rhythmical series will shift downward along its posterior slope, thus evoking primary reactions with decreased amplitude.

This supposition is easily tested by studying the temporal characteristics of the VEP developing against the background of the SN evoked by a second stimulus—in other words, by analyzing the recovery of the response to the third stimulus. Considering the shift of the SN summit, the theoretical prediction is that the A-potential of maximal amplitude must be obtained at intervals below 150 msec. The same reasoning holds for prediction of the VEP to the fourth stimulus delivered on the SN from the third, for the VEP to the fifth flash on the SN from the fourth, and so on. A study was designed to investigate peculiarities of the restoration of the reaction not only to the third, but also to the fourth, fifth, sixth, and seventh stimuli. The test flashes of light were presented at intervals from 50–220 msec after the preceding flash (Figure 3-2). Intervals between all

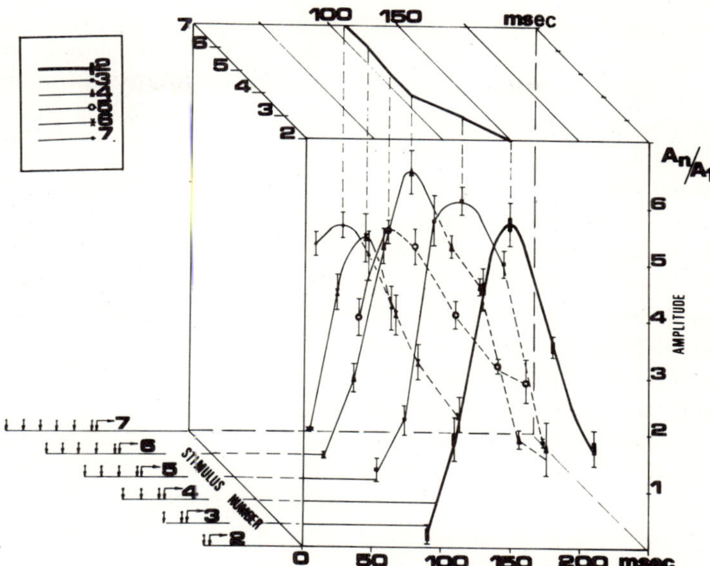

FIGURE 3-2. Family of curves reflecting the recovery of primary responses to the second through seventh light stimuli in a series. The response amplitude axis indicates the amplitude of the responses. The time axis shows the interval between the stimuli in milliseconds. The stimulus number axis indicates the ordinal number of the test stimulus. The arrows designate photic stimuli; their arrangement illustrates the experimental paradigm. Thus two arrows indicate that the first curve reflects the ordinary restoration cycle of the second response. The second curve is the restoration of the third response with two preceding light flashes serving as conditioning stimuli, and so on. The interval between conditioning flashes was 150 msec. A key (top, left) indicates each recovery curve from the second to the seventh. The curve on the top (the horizontal plane) of the three-dimensional graph shows the time to the maximum of each of the recovery curves. Note that all the recovery curves from the third through the seventh stimuli reach their maximum earlier than the initial recovery curve to the second stimulus. The axes of this graph are common with the stimulus number axis and abscissa.

flashes preceding the test stimuli were 150 msec. The restoration cycle of the last light flash was analyzed for each stimulus series, beginning with paired stimuli and proceeding sequentially to the series of seven flashes.

The family of curves obtained in the experiments are shown in Figure 3-2. They are characterized by a gradual decrease in amplitude, beginning with the third and ending with the seventh reaction, and by a gradual shift of the maximum recovery curves to the left. This concurs with the theoretical prognosis that the SN summit would seem to "slip away" from the stimulus. The effect is demonstrated even more convincingly by projecting the summit of every one of these curves to the top of the three-dimensional graph. The maximum of the curves, i.e., the exaltation phases, are clearly shifted to delays of less than 150 msec.

This experiment warrants the conclusion that aperiodic stimulation is required to obtain a series of A-potentials with stable amplitude. The duration of each interval in the series of stimuli should differ from the preceding one by a constant magnitude that equals the time shift of the SN summit to each stimulus of the rhythmic series.

It was possible to select these intervals by hand with the help of an oscillograph. The normal rhythmic response of the cortex to 7-Hz light flashes rarely consists of more than five A-potentials. Having at our disposal a stimulator designed to produce aperiodic series, we expected to be able to evoke a rhythmic response consisting of A-potentials of an approximately similar amplitude, i.e., sensory augmenting response without the waning phase. In any case, if our assumption was correct, the number of A-potentials should have noticeably exceeded the number in the ordinary rhythmic response of the cortex to periodic stimulation.

A special device was constructed to trigger an ordinary photostimulator. It appeared that it is possible to prolong the waxing phase with aperiodic stimuli but A-potentials stopped increasing after the fourth to fifth stimuli and maintained the amplitude attained for the fifth to the sixth flashes.

We could not present more than 11 stimuli in one aperiodic series because of the limitations of the technique. However, it was evident that the SN of the last response was somewhat diminished and the A-potentials displayed a tendency to wane. Although this type of stimulation made it possible to evoke a more synchronous response, it never led to abnormal activity during or after stimulation of any duration.

We compared the properties of aperiodic stimulation with those of regular intermittent light stimulation at any frequency and duration presented at any time of day. We concluded that an animal may be neurotized or blinded, but behavioral or electrographic fits cannot be induced in normal rabbits by any type of photic stimulation. This is indirect proof of the assumption that the brain must have some kind of abnormality for it to respond in the way specific to photogenic epilepsy. We were thus faced with the problems of identifying the nosologic specificity and the place of this abnormality in the family of epileptic diseases, and of deciding how to approach the study of its experimental model.

NOSOLOGIC SPECIFICITY OF ABNORMAL PHOTOGENIC REACTIONS

In 1944 Livanov used a method of rhythmical (3–4 Hz) stimulation using light flashes of increasing brightness. The stimulation was continued up to 5 sec, during which time the brightness was increased tenfold from subthreshold. The first changes in the EEG were used to determine the excitability of the cortex. Reactivity was appraised through changes in amplitude of activity. The type of driving response was categorized as *excitatory, balanced,* or *inhibitory.* This method was initially applied to Second World War veterans with occipital lobe injuries, with manifest or latent epileptic activity. Generally this type of stimulation activated or revealed abnormality. However, the probability of the activation of epileptic discharges varied for different types of driving responses. Discharges were intensified in the excitatory phases and inhibited or totally suppressed in the inhibitory phases (Livanov & Preobrazenskaya, 1947; Preobrazenskaya, 1945).

Perhaps now Livanov's method has but historical interest. But at that time his discovery of the activating potency of flickering light exerted the same influence in Russia as the study of Walter, Dovey, and Shipton (1946) did in Western clinical neurophysiology. It introduced the method of photic activation of epilepsy into clinical practice as an essential diagnostic of this disease.

Although photoepilepsy is the most frequent of the sensory precipitated epilepsies, it is encountered in only 2–4% of all epileptic patients (Bickford & Klass, 1969). According to Stevens (1962), 3% of the individuals who have focal epilepsy show EEG activation to flickering light, whereas 53% of patients who have generalized seizures and bilaterally synchronous 3-per-second W–S discharges show the same activation. In the absence of W–S complexes, but in the presence of diffuse abnormalities of electrocortical activity, a lowering of the photoconvulsive threshold is registered in 11% of all cases (Sellden & Hambert, 1968).

The number of patients sensitive to flickering light found by other researchers varies from 1.9% to 30–40% (Buchthal & Lennox, 1953; Melnitchuk, 1971; Melsen, 1958; Mundy-Castle, 1953; Schaper, 1957). These differences probably result from the heterogeneity of the groups of patients studied.

Melsen (1958) reported that 5.8% of epileptic patients who had a normal EEG exhibited the positive (abnormal) reaction to light. In the presence of focal lesions, abnormalities were found in 10.3%, and during diffuse pathology in 15%, of all cases. Activation was observed more frequently in women (13.9%) than in men (8.4%). The patients were regrouped according to the clinical manifestation of their seizures, and Melsen found that photogenic episodes emerged most frequently in petit mal epilepsy (32.1%) and in the combination of petit mal and grand mal seizures (25.8%). The greatest sensitivity to flickering light was registered in patients suffering from genuine epilepsy (19.7% of all cases in men and 29.7% of all cases in women). For symptomatic epilepsy these figures are correspondingly 6.8% and 6.6%.

A connection between photogenic seizures and centrencephalic pathology was also seen by other researchers (Naquet, Denavit, Lanoir, & Albe-Fessard, 1964; Niedermeyer, 1966). Most researchers have now concluded that up to one-third of patients having generalized forms of epilepsy display increased sensitivity to flicker.[1]

[1] Symposium on Epilepsy and Heredity, Paris (France), October 3, 1967. In *Epilepsia,* 1969, *10* (I).

Petit mal seizures are most frequently encountered in children, and it is thought that the frequency of photogenic reactions in children must be higher than in adults. Indeed, it was found that the child's brain is particularly vulnerable to flicker (Bickford, Daly, & Keith, 1953; Melsen, 1958). In 36% of children having behavior disturbances epileptiform discharges, generally W–S-type complexes, can be provoked. This figure increases to 68% if seizures are present in addition to behavioral disturbances (Mundy-Castle, 1953). Niedermeyer (1966) found that of those 0–20 years of age flicker caused clinical disturbances in 22%; in 76% it produced subclinical W–S discharges, multiple spike–wave discharges, or sharp and slow waves in the occiput. Examples of W–S discharges triggered in children who have photogenic epilepsy are shown in Figures 3-3 and 3-4.

Lerique-Koechlin, Nekhorocheff, and Le Mansec (1950) found pathological reactions to flicker in 32 of 90 children suffering from grand mal. In children

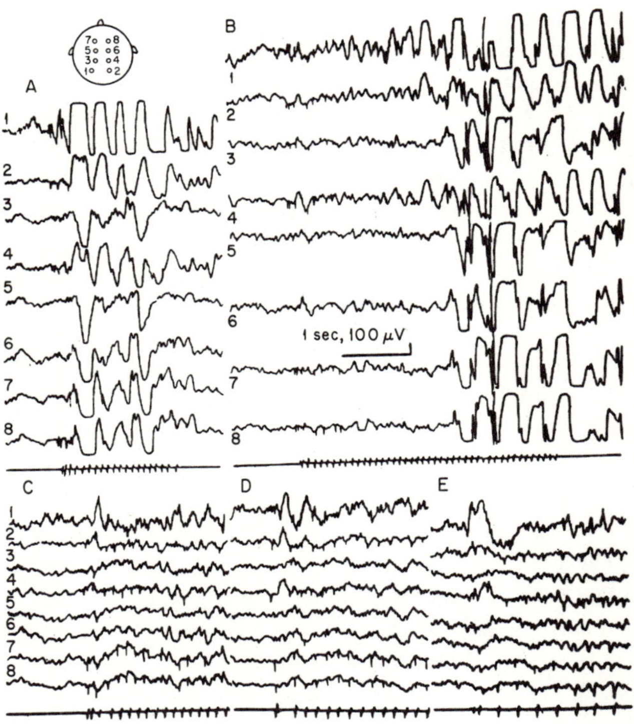

FIGURE 3-3. Examples of 3-per-second W–S discharges in patient L. K. Discharges were activated only by the flicker frequencies of about 12–15 Hz (A,B). Frequencies of about 9 Hz (C), 7 Hz (D), and 4 Hz (E) never evoked W–S discharges. Routine EEG examination. Binocular stimulation. Eyes closed. EEG electrodes are positioned in accord with the diagram in the upper left corner.

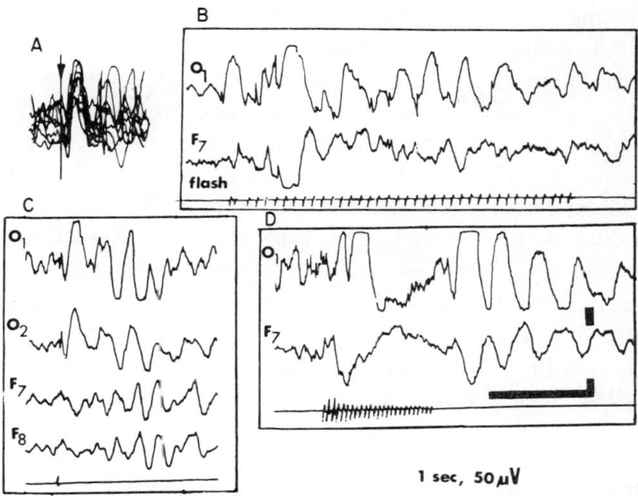

FIGURE 3-4. Wave—spike afterdischarges produced by a single light stimulus and by a short train of flickering light in the same patient (L. K.). Subject had eyes closed, binocular stimulation. A shows a high-amplitude visual evoked potential of wave—spike type recorded during routine EEG inspection and superimposed graphically. It is identical to the first components of W—S afterdischarges in the visual cortex. B shows a train of W—S discharges seen mainly under the left occipital (O_1) electrode. They are induced by 12-Hz intermittent light. C demonstrates W—S afterdischarge to a single photic stimulus. It is less pronounced in frontal (F) than in occipital leads. Such W—S afterdischarges are suppressed by a high-frequency flicker (D). Only the first stimulus of the train evokes a W—S discharge. Discharges reappear again after the cessation of stimulation (off-response). EEG electrodes are positioned according to the international 10—20 System.

having petit mal, photogenic reactions were found in 11 cases out of 26. Up to the age of 5 sensitivity to flicker is still comparatively low, but paroxysmal disturbances can be provoked by flicker at low frequency, about 3—8 Hz (Laget & Humbert, 1954). After the age of 5 sensitivity to light doubles.

Buchthal and Lennox (1953) reported that 1.4% of healthy children displayed a paroxysmal reaction to photic stimulation. There is, however, other information indicating that the number of such persons is much greater. Ulett and Johnson (1958) and Schaper (1957) found photogenic disturbances in 8.8% of their cases; Kooi, Eckman, and Thomas (1957) and Kooi, Thomas, and Mortenson (1960), in 4.1—6%; and Laget and Humbert (1954), in 7%. Therefore, the diagnostic value of light stimulation is much lower in children than in adults (Kiloh & Osselton, 1966). Most authors have found that activation of the hypersynchronous rhythm appears at frequencies from 8 to 20—25 Hz, which comprises the activation range (Bickford & Klass, 1969; Kiloh & Osselton, 1966; Melsen, 1958; Troupin, 1966; Watson & Bowker, 1965). Seizures and subclinical disturbances are observed most frequently at frequencies of 15—18 Hz but occasionally there are photogenic disturbances arising from flicker at a frequency far beyond the activation range.

In children of up to 5 years of age a seizure may be provoked by lower frequencies than in adults, and even by a single flash of light (Figure 3-4). Beginning at the age of 12 epileptiform disturbances may be provoked by the same frequency as at maturity. For this reason Livanov's reactivity curves can be used more successfully for the diagnosis of epilepsy in children.

Obviously in most cases photogenic seizures are petit mal seizures. Although in their pure form such phenomena are not frequent, their registration and consideration may help us to understand the general mechanisms of spontaneous seizures (Bickford & Klass, 1969). We should determine whether there is an elevation in sensitivity to intermittent light in any of the cases in which experimental W–S activity was produced in animals.

EXPERIMENTAL PHOTOEPILEPSY

An analysis of the pathological reactions to flicker was begun with the traditional study of the effects of Metrazol poisoning. I used a dose of Metrazol at which a single stimulus would evoke a series of W–S (EAD) discharges in normal awake rabbits.

Such discharges, as mentioned previously, generally emerge in patients having photoepilepsy during flicker or stimulation with paired photic stimuli, or as the aftereffect of intermittent light stimulation. The background EEG may be completely normal. The appearance of a series of W–S discharges in response to a single stimulus, similar to that demonstrated in Figure 3-4, is encountered relatively seldom. In cases where such reactions do take place, rhythmic light stimulation will undoubtedly provoke a photogenic seizure.

Contrariwise, following Metrazol poisoning true cases of photogenic epilepsy were the rare exception rather than the rule. This classification was restricted to bursts of a self-sustained paroxysmal activity, emerging in the course of light stimulation or as an aftereffect of flicker of varying frequency. However, complexes of the W–S type in response to a single stimulus and spontaneous bursts of paroxysmal activity were constantly registered in the EEG.

Stimulation by light at a low frequency (3–5 Hz) gave rise to rhythmic responses of a spike–wave form. An increase in the stimulation frequency to 6–10 Hz evoked unusually prolonged trains of sensory A-potentials, which together with portions of the SN looked like W–S evoked responses. Although both reactions possessed clearly expressed abnormal features, they were still driving responses, and there was no aftereffect following cessation of stimulation. When flicker of an even higher frequency (about 15–25 Hz) was presented, the series of W–S discharges (EAD) evoked by the first stimulus of the rhythmic series was not as readily suppressed by subsequent stimuli as in untreated animals. This resembled the activation of a burst of abnormal discharges.

Even without Metrazol injections the visual evoked potentials of animals frequently displayed patterns resembling W–S from the very beginning of low-frequency light stimulation. This looks like an abnormal response according to standards of the human EEG. Therefore specific criteria had to be established to determine experimental photoepilepsy. Three requirements were finally accepted:

1. W–S discharges must develop or continue after the cessation of flickering light of any frequency.
2. High-frequency flicker must lead to low-frequency W–S activity during stimulation.
3. Disturbances of consciousness should be associated with these episodes.

We encountered typical photoepilepsy in rabbits X-irradiated on the fifteenth day of embryogeny and in normal animals possessing lesions in structures of the limbic–reticular system. The reaction to flicker was studied in 26 X-irradiated rabbits. Generalized and bilateral W–S activity resembling genuine photoepilepsy was recorded in only 4, and it was almost exclusively evoked by high-frequency stimulation. It appeared during flicker and continued sometimes for about 30–40 sec after the cessation of stimulation (Figure 3-5). In 18 rabbits local W–S

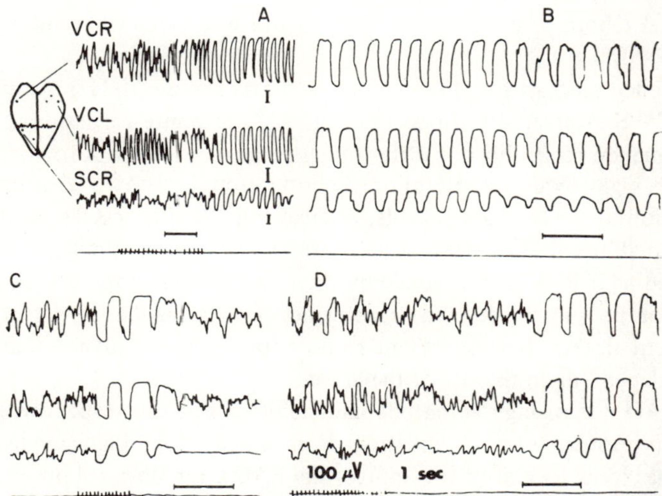

FIGURE 3-5. High-voltage, 2.5–3-per-second bisynchronous and generalized waves in rabbit, X-irradiated on the fifteenth day of embryogeny (dose 300 R). Freely moving animal with chronically implanted electrodes. Activity triggered by flickering light in A continued for 37 sec (continuation of A shown in B). In C and D are other examples of epileptiform discharges triggered in the same rabbit.

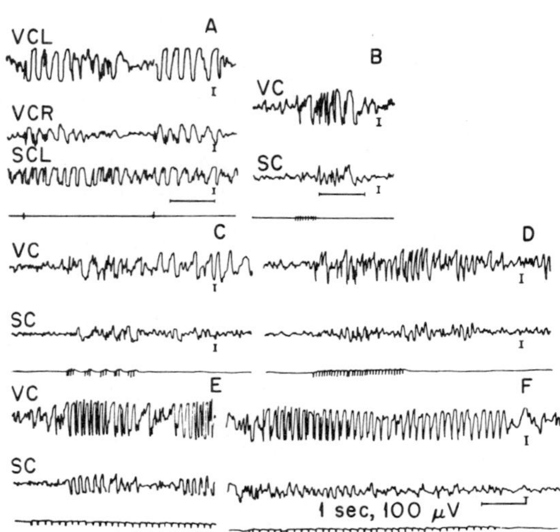

FIGURE 3-6. Different forms of the mildly abnormal electrocortical activity to light flashes (f) shown by rabbits X-irradiated on the fifteenth day of embryogeny. Note development of afterdischarges to, in A, a single light flash, and in B, C, and D, a rhythmical light flash. In E and F, prolonged spike–wave driving responses can be seen.

afteractivity was encountered in the visual cortex; prolonged sensory augmenting responses were also seen in rostral leads. The latter resembled the EEG response of normal rabbits after Metrazol injection but were somewhat more generalized (Figure 3-6).

In lesioned animals too, low-frequency flicker (below 10 Hz) practically never evoked W–S afteractivity. In general, the EEG response for lesioned animals in this frequency range did not differ much from that seen in X-irradiated rabbits. However, high-frequency intermittent photic stimuli activated W–S mostly during stimulation of the lesioned animals, whereas this occurred less frequently with the X-irradiated group. The effect usually started as soon as stimulation was begun. It seemed as if W–S EADs evoked by the first stimulus of the intermittent series could not be suppressed and transformed into a regular driving response by subsequent flashes. It is important to note for further discussion that this effect did not depend upon the site of the lesions.

The EAD was of high amplitude and stable and in this respect was similar to Metrazol photoepilepsy. I mentioned previously that high-frequency flicker sometimes loses its ability to suppress the EAD after Metrazol poisoning. But in lesioned animals the failure to suppress EAD was a consistent occurrence, and W–S discharges were sometimes of a lower frequency, approaching 3 per second, than those evoked by single flashes.

Both X-irradiated and lesioned animals differed from normal rabbits in their behavior during intermittent photic stimulation. When intermittent light stimuli of a low frequency (4–10 Hz) were presented to unrestrained normal animals they usually displayed orienting–exploratory behavior. With higher frequencies (more than 10 Hz) movements were more vigorous and resembled an avoidance reaction.

Lesioned and, especially, animals X-irradiated on the fifteenth day of embryogeny responded differently. If a flicker of any frequency was presented precisely *during* locomotor exploratory behavior, that behavior was terminated (probability .7).

It is probable that this arrest type of behavior is at least on the verge of what might be called an experimental photogenic petit mal fit. It is important to test this proposition in a more rigorous examination of behavioral response to flicker. The intent of the study to be discussed next was to test to what extent photoconvulsive responses of the W–S type block behavior and the integrative activity of the brain.

The experimental group contained four rabbits irradiated in midembryogenesis. Four groups served as controls. One control group consisted of four intact rabbits. Two others contained animals with electrodes implanted into various structures, which were subsequently destroyed. In one group, reflexes were elaborated before lesioning and a study was made of the effect of bilateral electrolytic injury in the zona incerta and the habenular nuclei. Animals were selected for the expression of photoconvulsive reactions. In the other group elaboration of conditioned reflexes was begun a week after electrolytic injury in the zona incerta and the habenular nuclei. The fourth group contained rabbits having injuries in various brain-stem areas that did not lead to the development of the W–S-type rhythm. This group consisted of rabbits treated according to the two control conditions described but who failed to show sufficiently expressed EEG hypersynchronization.

The conditioned stimulus was a 15-Hz flicker, which lasted for 15 sec. Current was passed as an unconditioned reinforcement through the floor grid of the experimental chamber 1–2 sec before the termination of flicker. To avoid shock the animal had to leave the start platform and enter a safe part of the chamber. If it made this response prior to the conditioned stimulus (*situational reflex*), it received a shock in the safe zone.

A study was also made of reaction to delayed reinforcement. Instead of increasing the delay of the unconditioned stimulus, the duration of the conditioned one was decreased. In this sense the term *delayed reinforcement* does not really describe the reflex. It is very difficult to establish classical trace reflexes in rabbits if the animal is required to avoid reinforcement *only* during the pause between the unconditioned and conditioned stimuli, and not during flicker. A genuine reflex in its adapted form was developed that fully satisfied the set task. We considered 9 correct responses out of 10 trials as the criterion for an established reflex.

Some 21 to 38 trials were required to establish a firm reflex in control animals. The animals left the start zone after 6.9 ± 0.8 sec. The distinction in the rate with which the reflex was established in the first two groups of control animals was not statistically significant. Transition to a delayed reinforcement (i.e., diminution of the time of flicker) exerted practically no effect on the latency of avoidance.

In irradiated animals the reflex was established after 29–56 trials. Two rabbits did not attain criterion even after 100 combinations. The remaining two rabbits showed virtually no difference from the control animals, except that they usually displayed a longer response latency (10.2 ± 1.3 sec). This delay was critical and the rabbits were sometimes subjected to painful electrical stimulation before they reached the safe zone.

Another essential difference in irradiated animals appeared when tests with delayed reinforcement were begun. Animals that had previously possessed a firm conditioned reflex displayed omissions of the reflex when the duration of flicker was decreased by 2–3 sec. Even after several hundred trials the reflex was always displayed with a probability of about .4. In three of the animals, even unconditioned avoidance was delayed; the animals often did not leave the start zone even after receiving a shock. The most paradoxical result in this series of experiments occurred when the duration of flicker was further shortened to 2–5 sec. In some animals the reflex was fully restored, or else its probability increased sharply.

Figure 3-7A shows an example of a normal conditioned reflex in an X-irradiated rabbit, which left the start platform 5–7 sec after the presentation of flicker. It can be seen that in irradiated animals there was no avoidance reaction to a flicker of shorter duration, and that the animals left the start zone only after receiving a painful shock (Figure 3-7B). The reflex was fully restored when the duration of flicker was further decreased (Figure 3-7C). The figure shows that the reflex was displayed following the first trial with the "new," shortened conditioned stimulus. The same result was obtained by random presentation of conditioned stimuli of varying durations. There were virtually no changes in the response after any number of trials.

The latency of avoidance to a very short conditioned signal varied, yet in this case, too, the animals just managed to avoid painful reinforcement. A firm conditioned reflex established in control animals prior to surgery disappeared completely following surgery if the unconditioned reinforcement coincided with the conditioned stimulus. Similarly, rabbits untrained before surgery did not learn the avoidance reflex to flicker after 100 trials (the probability of the reflex did not exceed .5–.6). But the reflex was successfully established in the control animals of the last group, who had received lesions that did not induce W–S activity. Therefore, the failures cannot be explained exclusively by nonspecific consequences of brain trauma or specific injuries, in definite brain structures, that disturb higher nervous activity.

FIGURE 3-7. Fragments of actographic records of avoidance conditioned reflex in X-irradiated rabbits with wave–spike afterdischarges to flickering light (experimental photoepilepsy). The flickering light was used as the conditioned stimulus. The unconditioned stimulus was electrical current (shock) delivered through the floor of the start platform (start zone). Time of avoidance to the safe zone was marked by a photocell when the animal crossed an infrared light beam. Numerals near the light channel indicate the total number of conditioning stimuli (CS) presentations (in parentheses) and the number of shortened CS presentations. A. Avoidance reaction undistinguishable from normal with a very short latency of the reflex unusual for X-irradiated animals with photoepilepsy. It was selected to show the avoidance of the normal type. B. Omission of the elaborated reflex after the presentation of shortened train of light stimuli. In this case it was the third presentation of this CS. Note that the rabbit moved into the safe zone only after the shock. C. Shows that this failure is not due to external inhibition since presentation of shorter train of light stimuli leads to the restoration of the reflex from the first presentation of the CS.

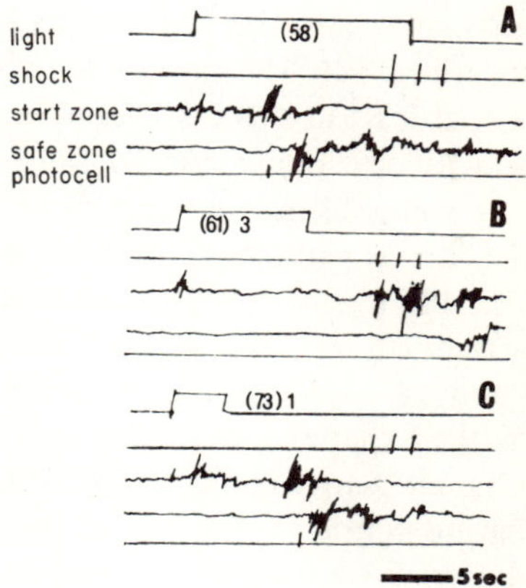

When the conditioned stimulus was shortened by several seconds, the conditioned reflex was restored in rabbits trained before surgery. Although its probability did not exceed .7, it should still be considered a true reflex. Most interesting, however, was the appearance of the reflex in rabbits of the third control group, in whom conditioning experiments were begun after surgery. They had left the start platform only episodically (probability .3), but the diminution in duration of the conditioning signal led to the appearance of the reflex with a probability of .8.

Let me now summarize the foregoing data:

1. Disturbance of learning in an avoidance reflex situation is not a nonspecific consequence of postirradiation or electrolytic brain injuries. It is, in fact, a dynamic disturbance manifested in certain specific conditions.

2. Neither can disturbances of conditioned reflex activity be explained by memory failures or difficulty in consolidating new material. The transition to delayed reinforcement restored the avoidance reflex, and this clearly shows that the animal had learned the problem but was unable to display the appropriate response.

3. A paradoxical improvement in the avoidance reaction was found in rabbits of the second and third control groups when the duration of flicker was shortened. At the same time a deterioration of the avoidance reaction was

observed in antenatally irradiated animals. In the latter case further diminution of flicker duration led to a restoration of the avoidance reaction.

It could be expected that changes in the parameters of the conditioning signal would lead to a deterioration of conditioned reflex activity through external inhibition. We observed an improvement of the reflex in some cases and a unique two-phase change in others, which indicated that the observed effects were associated with the bioelectrical brain reactions developing during flicker and in its aftereffect. The speed with which the reflex was established and its firmness are, at least in this case, functions of the expression and stability of paroxysmal activity developing in response to the conditioned stimulus.

It seems likely that this dependence does not only appear in conditions of deliberate pathology. In Chapter 1 attention was drawn to a delay in the "establishment" of the conditioned reflex in a rat having increased sensory afterdischarges. The word *establishment* has been placed in quotes because in the given case it was not so much the reflex of the animal that was being established as the experimenter's belief in the existence of the reflex. It was also noted in Chapter 1 that the reflex could not be established after dozens of trials in rats having injuries in the area of the habenular nuclei, but it unexpectedly appeared during EAD blockade. Thus, the effect does not necessarily result from an interruption of perception and memory mechanisms. It is more likely a difficulty in manifestation of an established temporary connection. However, as far as the experimenter is concerned, the manifestation of a reflex is synonymous with its existence, and a purely technical defect may lead to a false conclusion about complete blockade of integrative activity of the brain during experimental W–S discharges.

An attempt can be made to explain the reason for this unique disturbance of higher nervous activity in rabbits during the just-discussed series of experiments. Unfortunately, for technical reasons no EEG recordings were made during the behavioral experiment. Hence, all considerations are based on the EEG and the nature of the photoconvulsive reactions studied prior to the establishment of the conditioned reflex.

It seems that in animals with an embryonal radiation injury the reflex could be established as quickly as in intact animals in all cases. However, because of the hypersynchronization of the EEG during flicker, the reflex failed (was omitted) much more frequently than in intact animals. In two animals, possibly for the same reasons, criterion was never reached. Disturbance of the avoidance reaction in the second control group and the fact that it was "impossible" to establish the reflex in rabbits of the third control group can also be explained by the development of photoconvulsive reactions during the conditioned stimulus. Shortening of the duration of flicker enabled the rabbits in both control groups to leave the start zone. Long-lasting bursts of W–S-type complexes rarely developed in the aftereffect of flicker in these animals. It is likely that for this reason shortening of the action of flicker (delay of reinforcement) enabled the animals to *manifest the preliminarily established reflex.*

On the other hand, in antenatally irradiated animals the W–S discharges are expressed more clearly in the aftereffect of flicker than during flicker. The latter often desynchronizes the initial burst of W–S complexes. Therefore, shortening the duration of flicker leads to the development of hypersynchronous after-activity and the occurrence of an arrest reaction (an analog of petit mal), expressed by a dropout (omission) of the reflex.

Another circumstance of some interest is that the movement of irradiated animals into the safe zone proceeded with a somewhat longer latent period than in intact animals. Hence, a short pause between the conditioned and unconditioned stimuli allowed the developed afterdischarge to inhibit motor reactions. But with the minimum duration of flicker the hypersynchronous afterdischarge apparently ended before shock was administered, and in a number of cases the rabbit managed to enter the safe zone.

Naturally, this series of experiments can only be considered preliminary, and a final answer to all the questions posed will not be obtained soon. It will involve extensive analysis of various reflexes to flicker of different frequencies, taking into account the intervals between conditioned and unconditioned stimuli and, naturally, EEG activity.

ABNORMALITIES OF THE VISUAL CORTEX EXCITABILITY CYCLE AS A POSSIBLE CAUSE OF PHOTOEPILEPSY

The results presented in this section relate primarily to mechanisms of W–S activation during high-frequency stimulation. There is not only a question of why such a complex appears, but also why the SN is not fragmented by volleys of impulses evoked by the other stimuli of the rhythmic photic series. Since data on the peculiarities of the recovery cycle in normal rabbits have already been discussed in detail, I will directly describe excitability changes of the visual cortex in animals responding with abnormal reactions to intermittent light stimulation.

There is an important feature of the recovery cycle in X-irradiated and lesioned animals that makes the description and comparison of excitability abnormalities much easier. In animals exhibiting clear photoconvulsive reactions the recovery cycles are practically identical. This probably means that common pathogenetic mechanisms underlie experimental photogenic epilepsy in X-irradiated and lesioned rabbits.

Therefore, one animal having photogenic epilepsy episodes will be described as representative of the entire group. These episodes were the effect of injury in the areas of central gray matter and the habenular nuclei. The recovery cycle following Metrazol poisoning also has much in common with VEP restoration following injuries in the brain-stem area, but the latter models photogenic seizures far more accurately.

The main abnormalities in the restoration of the parameters of test responses can be predicted sufficiently from the observed increase in the amplitude and duration of the SN following brain-stem injury. In accordance with this prediction it was found that the absolute amplitude of the A-potentials considerably exceeded that in controls, and that they appeared with longer intervals between paired stimuli. The recovery curve in animals with photoepilepsy is not simply an exaggerated variation of the normal curve; distinct qualitative differences were found.

First, the restoration curve of the short latency (primary) potential amplitude (A_2/A_1) (Figures 3-1, 3-8) was steep and spike-shaped. This related to both the

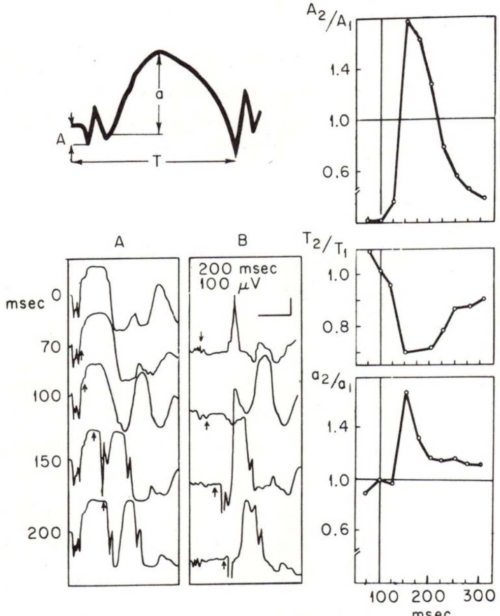

FIGURE 3-8. Peculiarities of the visual evoked potentials to paired stimuli and the restoration cycle of the test potential in rabbit with bilateral lesion in the habenular nuclei. Unanesthetized semirestrained rabbit, monocular stimulation. A. Averaged evoked potential to paired stimuli. Time between stimuli indicated on the left. Presentation of the first flash coincides with the start of the analysis; the second stimulus is indicated by an arrow. B. Differential tracings corresponding to each paired evoked potential in A except for the first (O delay) tracing. Note that with delays of 70–100 msec, the test stimulus does not evoke a separate response but hypersynchronizes the reaction to the conditioning flash. Potentials remaining in the differential traces show that the SN is broadened and afteractivity is facilitated. On the graphs: recovery of the primary potential (A_2/A_1), latency of the later response (T_2/T_1), and the amplitude of the SN (a_2/a_1). The ordinate indicates the parameter ratios; the abscissa indicates the interval between stimuli.

increase in amplitude of the A-potentials and an increase in the "refractory" periods. The potential to the test stimulus was small or absent when it was presented on the ascending slope of the SN and greatly attenuated when it fell on the descending slope. Sometimes responses were barely noticeable at intervals of 100–125 msec, when in normal animals this coincides with the exaltation phase.

Despite the absence of a separate response to a test stimulus delayed by 100 msec, the SN of the response to the first stimulus underwent certain changes. Growth of amplitude and duration was observed, the following LR increased sharply, and EADs emerged. This effect is better seen in the differential curve resulting from subtraction of the conditioning VEP from the summary reaction to paired photic stimuli (Figure 3-8). A high-amplitude negative potential remains in the record. In normal animals this is never observed, although it is sometimes found after Metrazol poisoning.

Another abnormality of the VEP parameter's recovery cycle was that diminution of the duration of the SN (see Figures 3-1 and 3-8) was less substantial than in normal animals, and to some extent this paralyzed the activity of the SN escape mechanism.

In other respects the VEP components to the second stimulus in lesioned and X-irradiated animals did not differ from those of normals.

In view of the data discussed previously on cellular response during the VEP, it is now possible to speculate on the nature of the abnormality leading to the increased sensitivity to flickering light of a high frequency. It can be deduced from the extraordinary facilitation of the duration and amplitude of the SN with closely spaced photic stimuli that the rhythmic stimulation leads to the summation of the inhibition underlying the SN and the SN is not replaced by a normal driving response pattern. This process should continue until the A-potential appears, initiating a new SN with the same properties. Thus, just this first complex may be viewed as the precursor of flicker-induced W–S discharges, which are simply SN (waves) and A-potentials (spikes). But I am anticipating; let us return to the description of normal and abnormal reactions of the visual cells to paired photic stimuli.

Excitability Cycle of Normal Cells

An analysis of the reaction of the visual cells to a paired stimulus showed that their responses depend on the type of short latency (primary) reaction as well as on the presence or absence of later discharges, coincided with the development of the LR. Thus, during short intervals between stimuli the most labile elements (i.e., those restoring their activity to the test stimulus most quickly) were cells excited during the following positivity of the primary response. On the other hand, intensification of firing during the A-potential was registered in cells responding to a single stimulus with later discharges.

Let me begin with the dynamics of the response to the second stimulus in cells that responded to a single stimulus predominantly with an initial discharge (Figure 3-9A). These cells did not respond to the second stimulus when presented at intervals from 50 to 80 msec. A second stimulus delayed for 100–110 msec evoked a consistent discharge. At intervals of 150–210 msec the initial discharge in these units became more regular but its probability was lower than in response to a single flash.

In cells that responded with initial inhibition-and-rebound discharges (Figure 3-9B), closely spaced stimuli (up to 80 msec) always produced an increase in the duration of the silence phase. This is also reflected in a shift of the maximum of the later response in the histogram. At intervals of about 110 msec the second stimulus started evoking episodic initial discharges that were not characteristic of

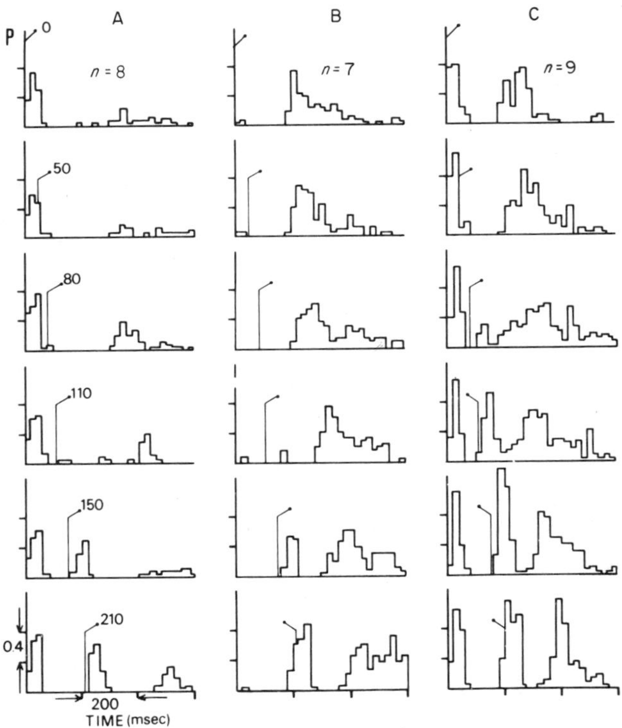

FIGURE 3-9. Averaging of discharges of normal visual units (PSTH) to double photic stimuli according to their type of response to a single flash (A,B,C). The ordinate indicates the probability of discharges (P). The abscissa shows the epoch of the response analysis in milliseconds. The presentation of the first flash coincides with the ordinate; the second stimulus is marked with a vertical line. The time interval between stimuli is given (in milliseconds), near the stimulus mark in A; *n* represents number of cells.

these cells. They finally formed a consistent short latency response when the test stimulus was delayed by 150 and 210 msec. This response was followed by a new inhibitory period and subsequent rebound. The inhibitory period to a test stimulus was always somewhat shorter than that to a single flash.

It would seem that the restoration cycle of cells responding with initial and later discharges should combine features of the cells described previously. However, these units showed certain peculiarities and were able to respond with minimal intervals between stimuli. A test flash presented at 80 msec evoked rather consistent spikes. By 110 msec short latency discharges appeared with the same probability as in response to a conditioning flash. With delays of 150 and 210 msec the short latency response became a powerful group discharge exceeding the probability of the firing to a single stimulus (Figure 3-9C).

Correspondingly, the first inhibitory period to the test stimulus in these units appeared when it was delayed exactly 80 msec. The duration of this second inhibitory period increased gradually with an increase in the separation of the stimuli, but it was always shorter than in response to a single flash. This was true even when the test stimulus evoked powerful short latency discharges. These inhibitory periods ended with a powerful rebound firing, thus indicating the IPSPs underlying the silent periods are probably highly synchronous and intense.

The seemingly paradoxical association of the shortened inhibitory period with powerful rebound discharges is perhaps explained by an increase in the physiological intensity of the second stimulus. Indeed, it was presented when the first stimulus had synchronized the most excitable low-threshold elements. Thus, the test stimulus had a rather favorable background for recruiting the response of additional units with higher thresholds. Taking into account that the magnitudes of the IPSPs of these cells are shorter, we can expect them to start rebound firing a bit earlier than the low-threshold population. This is a period when the IPSPs in most of the low-threshold elements can be overcome by synaptic depolarization, and as a result, the overall duration of the inhibition of the entire population will be shortened.

Evidently, the most visible changes of the cellular response appear when the stimulus is applied near the end of inhibition and prior to the regular LR. This occurs at a frequency of flicker of about 6–8 Hz (Figure 3-10). However, since these changes are closely linked with the emergence of A-potentials, they were evident when the typical spindle of the sensory augmenting response was developing. In 41% of the cases the emergence of A-potentials was accompanied by a distinct facilitation in the firing of the element. This was seen as an increase of the probability and frequency of discharge (Figure 3-10A,b); during SN fragments the usual suppression of action potentials was observed. During the waning phase of the spindles when the A-potentials were replaced by primary reactions of the ordinary driving response, there were fewer cellular discharges and impulse activity was often fully suppressed (Figure 3-10A,c).

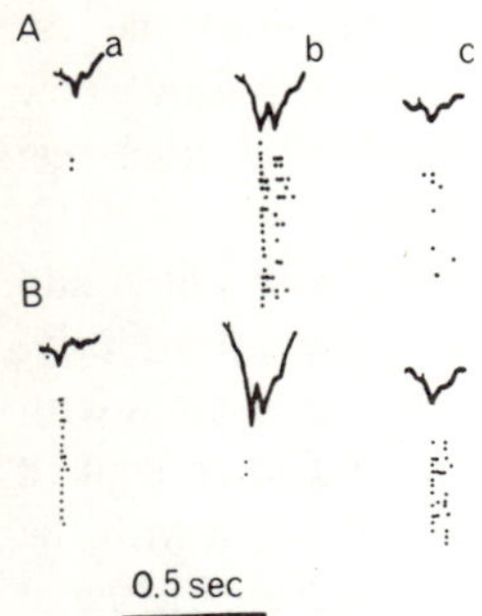

FIGURE 3-10. Raster dot display of two types of extracellular recorded spikes manifesting A, facilitation and B, suppression at firing during augmenting-type driving response: a, primary response and unit discharges to a single flash; b, augmenting potentials (A-potentials) of the waxing phase of the driving response; c, primary potential of the waning phase of the driving response. Photic stimulation frequency 7 Hz. Note that facilitation of unit activity during A-potentials is correlated with the suppression of firing during waning phase, and vice versa.

In 27% of the cells, however, it was precisely during the period of the emergence of A-potentials that the suppression of impulse activity took place (Figure 3-10B, b). This was renewed and even intensified when the A-potentials were replaced by primary reactions (Figure 3-10B,c). At 6–8-Hz stimulation the remaining 32% of the cells discharged episodically and in no connection with the summary reactions of the cortex, or they stopped their activity completely.

In the analysis of the excitability cycle of visual cells, some specific features were bypassed that relate to the formation of the initial cellular discharge in response to the test stimulus. Essentially, at that time we already had sufficient data to predict the nature of their rhythmic response. Figure 3-9C shows that cells reacting with early and later discharges to a single stimulus generate short latency discharges in response to a test stimulus at 150 or 210 msec. The frequency and probability of these discharges are much higher than those of the initial short latency spiking. Moreover, during this period initial firing appeared even in cells that normally respond to a single light flash with initial inhibition (Figure 3-9B). These cells increased their firing against the background of A-potentials. Contrariwise, cells that responded with inhibition during the A-potentials were frequently those that responded to a single stimulus with initial firing.

Naturally there are also transitory forms. Some responding with initial activation are at the same time able to join the group discharge during the emergence of A-potentials. It appears, however, that this takes place when they become able to respond with postanodal discharges. Mechanical injury to the unit by the microelectrode may create such a situation.

Thus, it can be assumed that the A-potential is the result of the summation of an intensified EPSP to a test stimulus and the rebound depolarization to the preceding stimulus. It is thought that for this reason the A-potentials and the LR have many properties in common (Myslobodsky, 1966). It can be concluded that if a cell shows the emergence of action potentials or an increase in their frequency during a series of A-potentials, it is a cell that responds with rebound discharges irrespective of the nature of the short latency discharge. The majority of visual cells respond in this way and therefore when a 6–7-Hz flicker is presented, 41% of the cells participate in the A-potential. During a gradual increase in the stimulation frequency cellular activity becomes less coordinated, and at 15–20 Hz or higher cells discharge sporadically, or else firing is totally suppressed.

Abnormal Excitability Cycle of Visual Cells

After Metrazol injection cell reactions similar to those in normals are registered, but in somewhat different proportions. There is a sharp decrease (up to 12.3%) in the number of cells reacting with tonic activation to a flash of light, probably related to an intensification of postsynaptic inhibition. And for the same reasons, there is also an increase in the number of cells reacting to the stimulus with initial inhibition (up to 43.4%). Elements reacting with initial and later discharges are encountered in 26.6% of all cases, and initial discharge alone was noted in 17.7%. We encountered a similar distribution of cells when analyzing the activity of rabbits antenatally irradiated in midembryogenesis. This could hardly be a coincidence. However, to be certain, it is essential to study the changes in spike activity of the same unit before and after Metrazol injection, and this was not done in the experiments described.

The most typical effect of Metrazol, as mentioned previously, is the development of cyclic activity in the cells. This is observed even during statistical analysis of cells that respond to a light stimulus predominantly with an initial discharge. During the presentation of paired stimuli, however, these cells react virtually as normals. The first indications of an initial response to a test stimulus were noted at delays of 90–110 msec. This is somewhat longer than for normal cells. When the second stimulus was delayed by 150 msec there was a sharp intensification of spike activity, but the probability of discharge did not match that to the first stimulus (Figure 3-11A).

Restoration of the activity of cells responding to a single stimulus with only a later reaction differed from normals in one way. During the presentation of a test flash at a delay of 60–90 msec a stable and regular increase in the duration of inhibitory pause was observed (Figure 3-12). This phenomenon is perhaps due to the summation of inhibition, and it is also frequently encountered in normal cells. But in the latter case cortical units that discharged during the short intervals between flashes could always be found. They could be regarded as initiators of the reactivation of hypothetical inhibitory interneurons, leading to the summation of inhibition. However, in photoepilepsy the presence of such reserve cells on the cortical level seems unlikely, because of the hypersynchronization of activity.

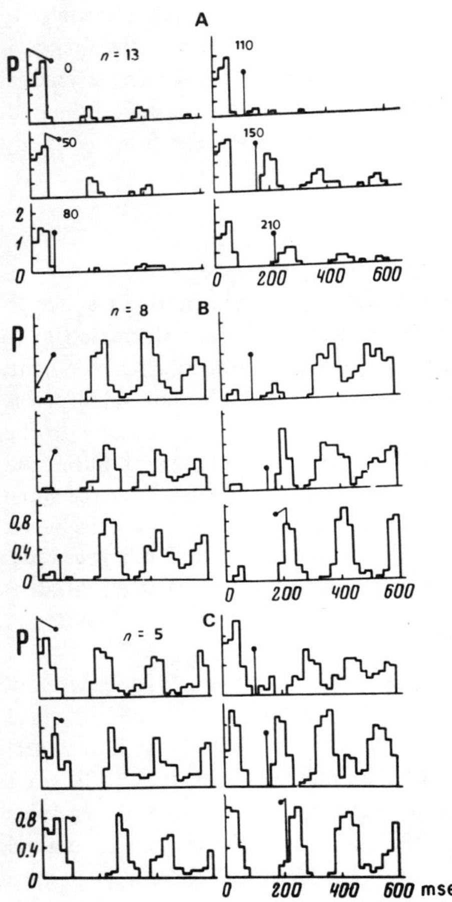

FIGURE 3-11. Averaged unit discharges for different types of units (A,B,C) to double photic stimuli after intravenous Metrazol injection. Note the typical picture of phasing of neuronal discharges. For details of description see Figure 3-9.

The hypersynchronization of cell reactions, evoked by the conditioning stimulus, can be proved by an extremely simple method. Figures 3-12 and 3-13 show the same poststimulus time histograms we saw in Figures 3-9 and 3-11. The difference is that in Figures 3-12 and 3-13 the histograms are superimposed. In the first case (A) the ordinate (frame of reference) coincides with the first stimulus (test stimuli are marked by arrows), whereas in the second case (B) the frame of reference coincides with the presentation of the test stimulus. Clearly, the latter method of analysis holds the only possibility of revealing the characteristic patterns of the restoration of cell reactions. Normally other methods of analysis would lead to disintegration of the histogram. It assumes an unnaturally extended form (Figure 3-12B), because there is no coincidence in the timing of the emergence of the reaction.

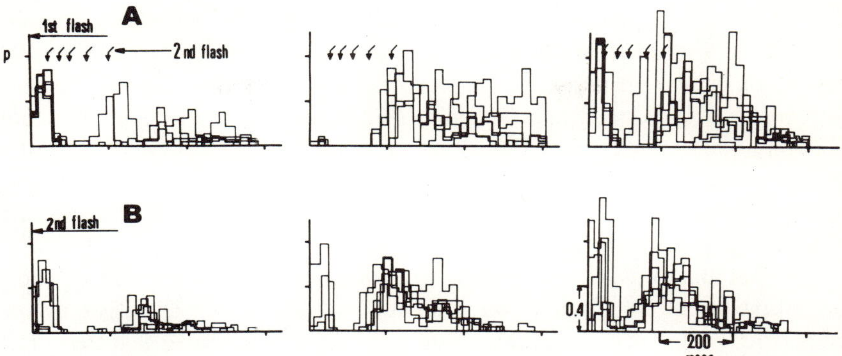

FIGURE 3-12. The same PSTHs as in Figure 3-9. All PSTHs are superimposed according to the type of cell discharges, though intervals between flashes were ignored. In A is shown the superimposition of graphs, with the first stimulus serving as a frame of reference. The second stimuli are marked by arrows. In B is shown the superimposition of graphs, with the second stimulus serving as a frame of reference. Note that only in B are PSTHs clearly spatially coherent.

Following Metrazol injection, the superimposition of the poststimulus time histograms referenced to the first stimulus usually fully preserved the normal picture of reaction to a single light flash (Figure 3-13A). But when referenced to the second flash, the characteristic pattern of the reaction grew more obscure (Figure 3-13B).

It seems that under these conditions the first stimulus evoked activation of an enormous number of cells, probably close to the maximum. Hence, the second stimulus was unable to overcome the synchronized inhibition of the majority of

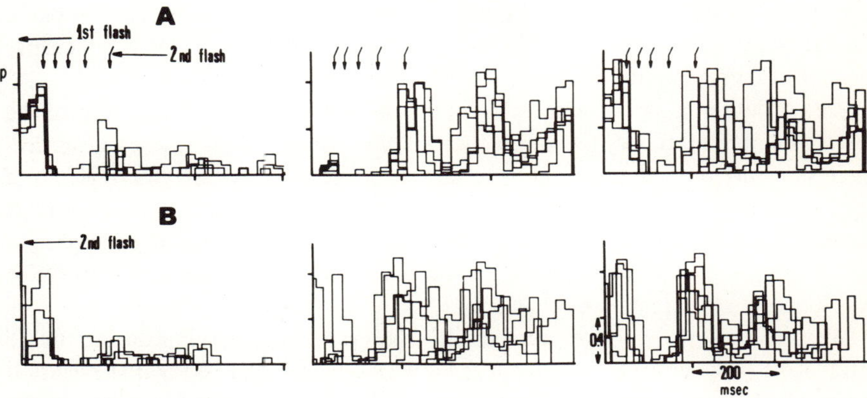

FIGURE 3-13. The same PSTHs as in Figure 3-11, after intravenous Metrazol injection. They are superimposed (as in Figure 3-12) according to the type of cell discharges. The frame of reference is the first (A) or the second (B) stimulus. Note that after Metrazol poisoning one may see PSTH coherence in A.

the cell population and to induce them to discharge. The test photic stimulus can reactivate a new inhibition–discharge cycle only when presented near the end of the inhibition period to the conditioning stimulus. Following Metrazol poisoning the poststimulus histograms, referenced to the first stimulus, look much more coherent because the second stimulus is unable to affect the initial response. For the same reason the response referenced to the second stimulus produced histograms that are not coherent. The test stimulus evokes cell reactions in a narrower range of delays than normally.

I feel that due to the current paucity of data it is premature to speculate about the nature of the net that allows summation of inhibition. There is only one remark that seems relevant in this context. I have already noted that the cortex is the first to be drawn into the hypersynchronous rhythm following Metrazol injection. Although the LGB elements may participate in the organization of the W–S rhythm, this is not accompanied by excessive synchronization of the LGB activity. The latter is only drawn into W–S-type rhythm at the stage of rather severe poisoning. It is quite likely that the reserve (nonhypersynchronized) cells, able to discharge a second time at the presentation of a closely spaced second stimulus or during high-frequency intermittent photic stimulation, are located in the LGB. This warrants the assertion that the channel of afferent inhibition may be made up of the axons of relay cells.

A preliminary analysis conducted in X-irradiated rabbits with experimental photogenic seizures revealed clearer summation of inhibition in visual cells under the same conditions of stimulation. As shown in the poststimulus time histogram (Figure 3-14) based on the analysis of the visual cell activity in rabbits X-irradiated in midembryogeny, the inhibitory pause increases even during presentation of the test stimulus 100–120 msec after the conditioning one. Judging from the latent period of the later discharge, the duration of the inhibitory pause increases by 30 msec or more (36.8 ± 7.6 msec), which correlates satisfactorily with the corresponding increment in SN duration in these animals (43.1 ± 2.2 msec). In other respects these cells are similar to normal cells. Hence, unlike the effect of pure Metrazol, the summation of the inhibition here is clearly noticeable not only in analysis of the reactions of single cells, but also as reflected in the summary VEP. It may be that the channel of afferent inhibition, whose function was suspected from studies of Metrazol poisoning, is under the control of structures of the limbico–reticular complex, and that their injury removes or weakens these restraining mechanisms.

We can now attempt to "reconstruct" the events that develop during flicker and lead to the activation of epileptiform W–S-type discharges. Light stimulation of 6–10 Hz leads to progressive synchronization of the electrical activity of the normal cortex, because of the recruitment of new elements. This process prepares the high-threshold cells and later draws them into the reaction. The duration of IPSPs of the latter and, hence, the frequency of their pulsation may

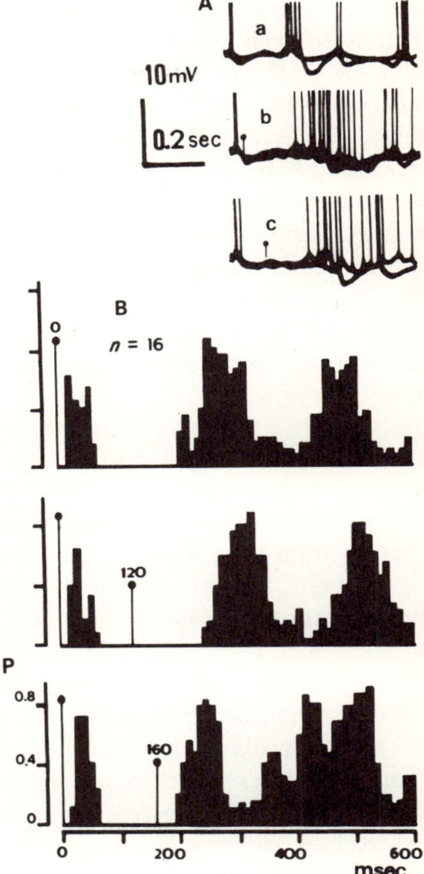

FIGURE 3-14. Prolongation of inhibitory period in neurons of the visual cortex by the second flash presentation. A. Superimposed tracing of quasi-intracellular recording of the cellular responses to a, single, and b and c, double stimuli. Second stimulus is marked by a dot. Number above the dot indicates the separation between stimuli. B. PSTHs to single and paired flashes of 16 extracellularly recorded cells. Middle PSTH demonstrates consistency of the effect shown in b and c. Unanesthetized immobilized rabbit X-irradiated on the fifteenth day of embryogeny. Metrazol (3 mg/kg) was injected to stabilize the wave–spike pattern. Ordinate indicates the probability of the cellular discharges. Abscissa shows the epoch of the response analysis in milliseconds.

differ considerably from the oscillations of most of the elements in the more active part of the cell population. It is also likely that because of their higher threshold, they respond with shorter IPSPs. The premature completion of inhibition in this micropopulation and the appearance of earlier rebound discharges will shorten the duration of the IPSP of other elements, and according to the model of Andersen and Andersson (1968) this limits the synchronization from light stimulation.

In X-irradiated, lesioned, and Metrazol-poisoned animals the spontaneous appearance of W–S (SEAD) discharges testifies to higher initial synchronization of cortical activity. Indeed, the amplitude of the SN of the test response depends on both the expression of the SN to the conditioning stimulus and the amplitude of the short latency reaction to the test flash. The test IPSPs emerge against an initially hyperpolarized background, but owing to their collateral activation, they also depend on the parameters of the initial cell discharge. Correspondingly, if all other conditions are equal, the probability of an initial discharge will vary with the amplitude of the SN. This dependence is equally well preserved in normal as well as operated animals. In the latter, however, the a_2/a_1 and tg_2/tg_1 curves (Figures 3-1 and 3-3) are generally on a lower level, which probably indicates that the possibility of further synchronization of the activity of these elements has already been exhausted (Myslobodsky, 1970c, 1971). Hence, it may be assumed that with every new stimulus of the rhythmic series fewer new cells are drawn into the reaction than in normals. The mechanisms for changing the SN parameters are accordingly restricted; they proceed more slowly. In lesioned and irradiated animals the reaction to low-frequency light stimulation following Metrazol poisoning acquires the characteristic shape of very durable spike–wave spindles.

Practically, in Metrazol-treated or X-irradiated animals, as well as in normal rabbits, low-frequency stimulation reproduces the same process, which proceeds with the frequency of spontaneous activity. The gradual recruitment of the new cells into this reaction leads at a certain stage to the desynchronization of the response, thus preventing the development of self-sustained W–S activity. This assumption is supported by the fact that the cellular structure of the low-frequency driving response in X-irradiated animals or after intravenous Metrazol injection does not essentially differ from that in normal rabbits (Myslobodsky, 1970a). Clear differences are encountered only during high-frequency flicker.

When presenting high-frequency flicker to normal animals, we desynchronized the SN and evoked a low-amplitude rhythmical response, which consisted of primary responses or their components, i.e., of low-amplitude EPSPs. Because of the summation of inhibition, during high-frequency stimulation, X-irradiated and lesioned animals evinced a paroxysmal increase in the SN amplitude and duration instead of its desynchronization, and this was maintained until the rhythmic avalanche attained its maximum. As a result a new "A-potential–SN" complex appeared and the cycle repeated. Naturally, this type of activation requires the presence of the SN, and therefore often emerged at the very beginning of stimulation. There were also relatively frequent cases of the appearance of the SN in the course of stimulation by high-frequency flicker.

We have the impression that prolongation of the inhibitory period is the factor that leads to the urgent hypersynchronization of cellular activity and creates the basis for W–S activation by high-frequency flicker.

4 Clinicophysiological Approach

LIMITS OF THE PHYSIOLOGICAL VARIABILITY OF EVOKED POTENTIALS OF THE HUMAN BRAIN

According to the extensive data found in the literature, the human visual evoked potential (VEP) is a low-amplitude polyphase complex that ends in an alpha afterdischarge. No single component of this response is comparable with the VEP waves in the visual cortex of animals, with the possible exception of primates, the VEP of which has not been studied extensively. In addition the numbers and letters used to label VEP components have created the illusion of some exclusiveness of that response, of the individuality and independence of its waves. True, there seems to be a consensus of opinion among most researchers that human VEP has primary and secondary components. However, it is not known at what level of oscillation (in a series of highly similar waves) and according to what criteria such a division should be made. Besides, the attempts to find primary and secondary components are made to reveal the relative specific and nonspecific contributions to the organization of the VEP, since the sequence of bioelectrical events in response to a stimulus implies their genesis. This terminological nuance suggests a decrease in the degree of the specificity of VEP components with increasing latency. This becomes a major obstruction when a study is made of the VEP of humans; there are no helpful analogies, and the possibility of experimental analysis is limited.

We thus encounter two possibilities:

1. The assumptions advanced in the preceding sections do not extend to man. The organization of "spontaneous" hypersynchronous rhythms and photo-convulsive reactions proceeds according to principles distinct from those operating in the rabbit.
2. The mechanisms of hypersynchronization of the EEG in humans and animals are the same; but in humans and primates a certain superstructure that stabilizes their reactions and camouflages the precursors of abnormal rhythms has evolved.

If the first assumption is correct, it is essential to disclose the distinguishing features in the organization of spontaneous and evoked paroxysmal reactions in humans. If, on the other hand, the second assumption is correct, we may succeed in revealing the precursors of convulsive rhythms in epileptics, and this should unmask the preformed mechanisms. Besides, for seizures to emerge some conditions, such as a definite age or state of consciousness, must exist. These perhaps also evoke changes of the response in normals in the same direction as pathology.

A Few Words about the Method

The following experiments were conducted with the subject reclining in a special armchair in a dark, screened, soundproof room. Occipital electrodes were placed an inch higher and an inch to the outside from the inion on both sides. The other electrodes for the registration of the routine EEG and for the episodic registration of VEPs from the more rostral areas were placed according to the "10–20" international system. Linked mastoid electrodes served as reference.

Routine EEG, electromyogram, and oculogram were registered and amplified by a 17-channel Nihon-Kohden EEG machine. In most cases it was found that averaging 25–30 reactions was sufficient to obtain a stable and reproducible VEP. The use of a larger number was undesirable, since the state of the brain, especially in patients, is rather unstable. As a result, the VEP obtained using more than 30 reactions could be a reflection of the brain reactivity during greatly varying spans of time, which would be physiologically and pathophysiologically senseless.

The time to the maximum and the amplitude (from peak to peak) of all VEP components, the latent period, the frequency and time of the increment of the sensory alpha-afterdischarge (SAD), and the asymmetry coefficient of the VEP of both hemispheres were all statistically processed.

The strobe was placed 20 cm from the bridge of the nose. The flash energy was 0.3 joules, its duration 150 μsec (stimulators Nihon Kohden, RFT, and Bio-fizpribor). The interval between flashes did not exceed 3 sec. Stimulation was usually aperiodic. The stimulus was accompanied by an audible click, which, however, did not evoke a visible potential at the occiput.

The subjects were healthy persons of both sexes, from 6 to 15 and 19 to 30 years of age. (The second group included mainly students and my colleagues.) All had normal or corrected vision.

General Characteristics of the VEP to a Single Stimulus

The VEP of a waking relaxed subject sitting with closed eyes generally begins with a negative wave that reaches its maximum after 40–50 msec. In about 20% it is preceded by a low-amplitude positive oscillation with a latent period on the order of 25–30 msec. Following the negative or positive–negative oscillation, three more positive–negative complexes develop. To obviate difficulties, we shall for the time being also label the latter according to their polarity (letters) and sequence (digits). A typical average VEP is illustrated in Figure 4-1; the time to maximum and the amplitude of each of its waves are shown in Table 4-1. The table does not give the characteristics of the fifth positive wave. It is singled out by some authors; however, our experience indicates that it is not a "response per se," but an oscillation of the sensory alpha-afterdischarge (AD) and its identification is rather arbitrary.

AD appeared in the occipital derivations with a latency of 304.40 ± 5.51 msec (time to the peak of the first negative oscillation). Its frequency fluctuates between 8 and 12 per second (11.4 ± 0.23 per second), depending on the frequency of the alpha rhythm. Its amplitude depends greatly on the degree to which it is expressed. Naturally, in the rostral and temporal derivations the AD is

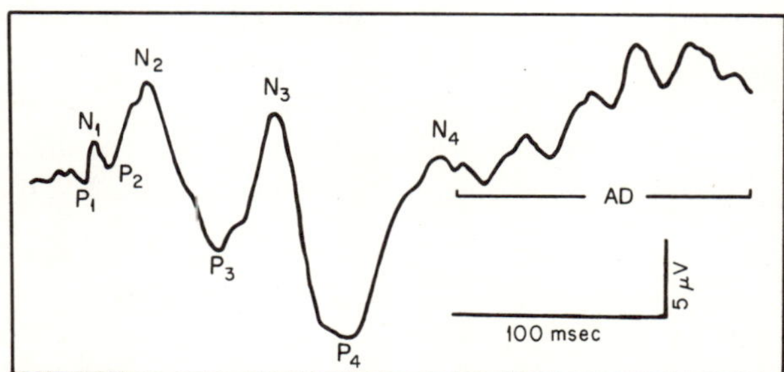

FIGURE 4-1. Example of the typical averaged VEP. Letters and numbers identify wave components according to their polarity and sequence. AD represents alpha-afterdischarge. Healthy, waking female subject with eyes closed. Here and in all subsequent figures active electrode on the right occiput referenced to linked mastoids. Negativity in this and in all subsequent tracings is indicated by an upward deflection. This averaged trace is based on 30 stimulus presentations. Only during sleep studies and in epileptic patients was the number of stimulus presentations reduced to 20–25. Here and in all subsequent evoked potentials record analysis commences with stimulus onset.

TABLE 4-1. Peak Latency and Peak Amplitude of Components of Averaged VEP in Healthy Subjects (Mean ± Standard Error)[a]

VEP components	Peak latency (msec)	Amplitude (μV)
P_1	36.0 ± 0.62	1.8 ± 1.05
N_1	43.4 ± 0.77	9.4 ± 1.09
P_2	60.7 ± 1.45	8.5 ± 1.04
N_2	77.5 ± 1.84	12.8 ± 1.60
P_3	106.5 ± 2.55	21.7 ± 2.32
N_3	129.4 ± 3.76	13.2 ± 1.98
P_4	167.4 ± 4.11	22.5 ± 2.87
N_4	217.2 ± 6.55	22.0 ± 2.36

[a]All statistical analysis were performed on data on 32 subjects. P_1 parameters calculated in 6 subjects.

practically absent. However, in people with fairly abundant alpha and in conditions of quiet wakefulness bordering on drowsiness, it can be seen in the rostral derivations.

The data on the form and parameters of the VEP coincide, in the main, with other studies using comparable techniques of recording, stimulation, and analysis of electrical reactions (Dustman & Beck, 1965; Kooi & Bagchi, 1964).

VEPs generally maintain their form during changes in the direction of attention and have a similar composition irrespective of the location of their registration (Kudinova & Myslobodsky, 1970).

Naturally, however, the parameters of individual waves may differ considerably in the different derivations. If photic stimulation is presented while the subject's eyes are open, the VEP changes considerably, mainly because of the emergence of a slow negative wave (SN) or the suppression of the AD, as shown in Figure 4-2. Judging from the time to the maximum of the SN, it evolves from

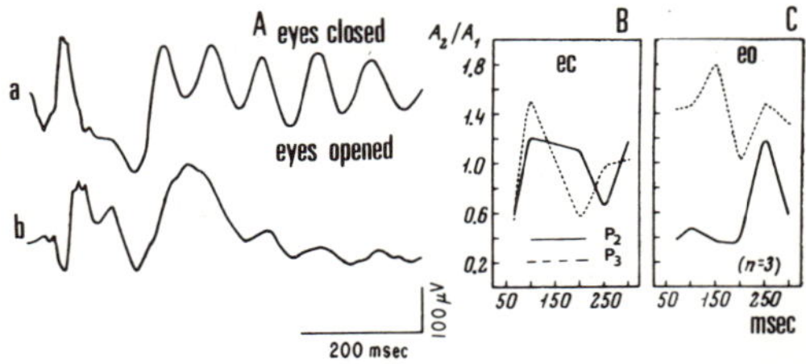

FIGURE 4-2. Comparison of A, evoked potentials and B, C, the recovery function during stimulation in b, eyes opened and a, eyes closed conditions. In graphs B and C, the ordinate indicates the ratio of the amplitudes of P_2 and P_3 waves to the test stimulus. The abscissa gives the intervals between paired stimuli. The data have been averaged from three subjects.

the fourth negative oscillation. This assumption is also confirmed by an analysis of cases where AD is depressed without so steep an increase of the N_4 wave, as shown in Figure 4-2. Further support comes from the metamorphosis of the VEP during sleep, of which more will be said later. The waves P_4 and N_4 are the only components whose peak latency and duration increase for 10–20 msec when the eyes are opened. The time to the peak of all other VEP waves decreases by 5–20 msec. The most characteristic changes of amplitude are displayed by wave P_2, which increases noticeably, and by waves N_2 and P_3, which are generally reduced (Myslobodsky, 1970a, 1971). As was discussed previously, Kudinova and I found that opening the eyes only suppresses the SAD if the eyes are focused on the light source or if the eyeballs converge maximally (when the subject tries to look at the tip of his nose). An upward or maximal lateral deviation of the eyes in the direction habitual for a subject restored the AD (see Figure 4-3A) although the strobe was always located in the visual field (Kudinova & Myslobodsky, 1970).

There were even more demonstrative experiments in which the subject accommodated his eyes on an imaginary or real distant fixation point (see Figure 4-3B). The AD, which had formerly been fully suppressed, appeared whenever the strobe was removed from the field of clear vision. True, it did not attain its initial amplitude and was generally smaller than the AD emerging during maximum deflection of the eyes. However, judging from the subjects' self-observation and reports, their gazes almost unavoidably shifted periodically toward the strobe. It is important to note that in all such cases the AD was clearly

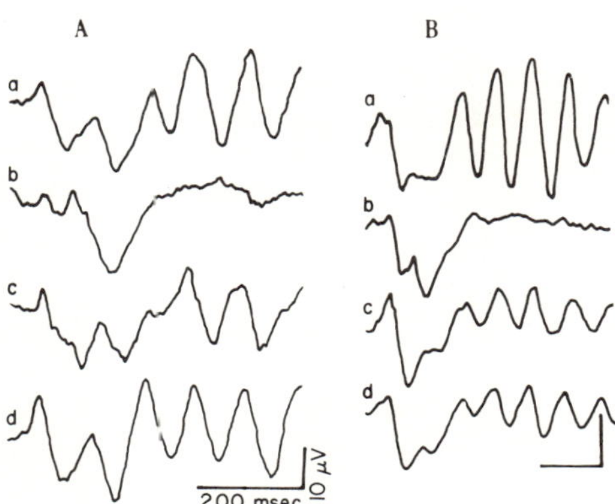

FIGURE 4-3. Influence of A, eye positions and B, lens accommodation on the alpha afteractivity of the evoked potential in different subjects. Background potential with prominent afteractivity in eyes-closed state (a) in A and B. In both cases afteractivity is suppressed in the eyes-opened state with fixation on the strobe (A,b and B,b). Upward (A,c) and lateral eye-shift (A,d) fixation on a very dim test-object 2 m behind the strobe (B,c), concentration on an imaginary fixation point after the switching-off of a real one (B,d). All these tests led to resumption of the alpha afteractivity. Calibrations for A: 100 msec, 10 μV; for B: 200 msec, 10 μV.

expressed, even though photic stimulation was presented to open eyes and following these instructions required a definite effort. Functions of the reticular formation were undoubtedly activated. These results also acquire interest if it is borne in mind that the position of the eyes is important to the organization of convulsive activity, especially in cases when it emerges in response to eye closure (Green, 1968), or when a seizure sets in during random blinking. This effect cannot be attributed exclusively to changes in the illumination of the retina or to photic flicker produced by blinking, since seizures of this type can set in in complete darkness. It seems probable that in both cases there is some link between voluntary eye movements and the hypersynchronization of electrical brain activity. The eyes turn upward during closure and move slowly in the same direction during blinking. It may be that some pathology of the oculomotor system plays an important role in the pathogenesis of photogenic epilepsy.

Because it is an alpha derivative the AD should change greatly when the direction of visual attention is changed. However, the result obtained was not in good accord with this prediction. Data summarized in Table 4-2 show that when the subject's attention was attracted to photic stimulation the AD amplitude was depressed by 20–25%. This occurred when the subject was instructed to count the flashes or detect differences in their brightness (the brightness of the flash remained unchanged). At the same time the AD amplitude did not decrease and was sometimes even exalted when the subject was required to press a lever in response to each flash, although in some cases he was instructed to count the flashes simultaneously. Because of the great variability of data both during quiet wakefulness and during the execution of instructions, these results were not

TABLE 4-2. The Influence of Attention Changes on the Alpha-Afteractivity Parameters (Mean ± Standard Error)[a]

	Alpha-afteractivity parameters			
Series	Peak latency (msec)	Frequency (per second)	Amplitude (μV)	Steepness (derivative of the envelope)
Counting of stimuli	311.0 ± 5.97	12.8 ± 0.29*	13.1 ± 1.46	1.8 ± 0.45
Motor response to stimuli	316.1 ± 7.18	12.6 ± 0.3*	15.8 ± 1.99	1.5 ± 0.37
Problem solving	307.0 ± 12.15	12.1 ± 0.49	17.1 ± 2.86	2.5 ± 0.95
Programmed motor activity	308.4 ± 7.29	11.6 ± 0.26	17.6 ± 2.25	2.7 ± 1.4
Background	304.4 ± 5.51	11.4 ± 0.23	17.6 ± 2.27	2.0 ± 0.33

[a]All statistical analyses were performed on data of 19 subjects.

*$p < .001$.

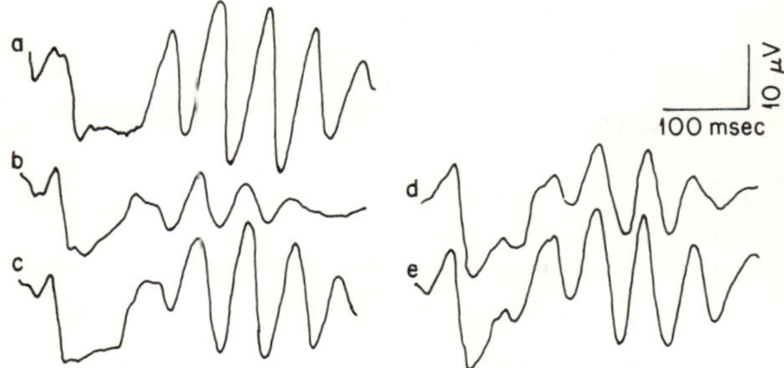

FIGURE 4-4. Changes of afteractivity of VEPs during shift of attention. Subject's eyes closed. Relaxed state (a). Distraction of the subject's attention from the stimulus was attained by having the subject solve a mathematical problem (b) or operate a switch according to a complex program of fine hand movements (c). Attraction of the subject's attention to the stimulus was attained by having the subject count the total number of flashes or select the number of "dim" stimuli (d) or press a switch in response to every flash (e). Note that afteractivity is facilitated during c while waves P_3 and P_4 are selectively potentiated when the subject attends to stimuli (d,e).

statistically significant when averaged for the whole group. However, individual results (Figure 4-4) were so accurately reproducible that I consider the fact worth mentioning.

Further, when the subject was asked to solve simple mathematical problems to distract his attention from stimulation, the AD was somewhat depressed. It reappeared however, and in some experiments its amplitude even exceeded initial value, when attention was distracted by the performance of a comparatively complex program of hand movements.

Distraction of attention requires that the subject concentrate on some other task which in this case is complex enough to induce arousal. But at best, the AD amplitude remained at the same level as during quiet wakefulness (Figure 4-4). Changes of the P_3 and/or P_4 components in this experiment were similar to those described by Lindsley and discussed previously. They were usually somewhat facilitated when the subject's attention was focused on external photic stimuli (Spong, Haider, & Lindsley, 1964).

The AD was particularly increased during execution of a motor task, irrespective of whether the subject gave special attention to the number and character of the stimuli (Figure 4-4). Figure 4-5 shows the other fragment of this experiment, which Kudinova and I made to determine the influence of periodical and aperiodical fine hand movements on the AD amplitude. This experiment revealed that eye movements grew more distinct with the beginning of fine hand movements (Figure 4-5C,D). It should be noted that in this case there was a clear facilitation of the AD of the VEP (Figure 4-5D) ($p < .01$), returning us again to the problem of eye movement and alpha rhythm.

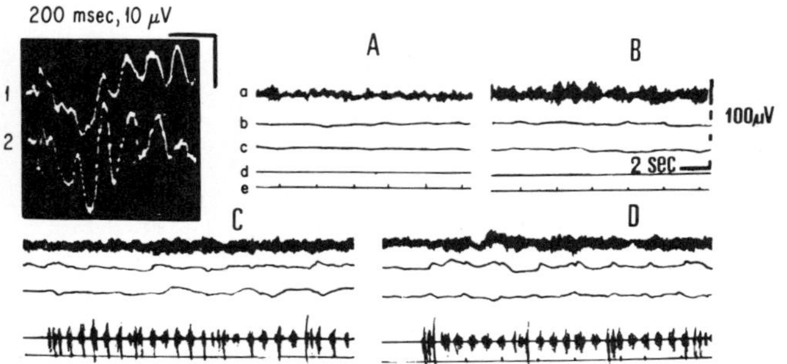

FIGURE 4-5. Ocular movements and alpha afteractivity of the VEP. Fragments of a, EEG; b and c, EOG; and d, EMG during resting condition with eyes A, opened and B, closed. Light stimulus mark in e. In D the switch was pressed according to a program with eyes closed. In C the subject pressed a switch in response to a flash. Visual evoked potentials 1 and 2 were recorded during B and D conditions, respectively. Note facilitation of the afteractivity in 2.

The data described here are in agreement with those of Mulholland and Evans (1966) and Dewan (1967), which demonstrated that alpha may partially depend upon the position of the eyes and lens accommodation. However, recalling the discussion on the nature of alpha, I have to note that the data do not support Lippold's theory (1973) that the alpha rhythm is an artifact resulting from eye movements. At least as far as interpretation of the data is concerned, I feel all these facts are merely revealing the general principle that brain structures participating in the organization of a certain rhythm (or rhythms) may be partly controlled by manipulating the state of the peripheral organs, be it eye movement or general muscle tonus. These data show how many variables must be controlled to be certain that VEP abnormalities can be considered a consequence of a definite brain pathology.

The VEP to Light in Children. The specificity of the responsiveness of the child's brain to photic stimulus was studied in children aged from 6 to 15 years. This is the age period when, according to a number of researchers (Creutzfeldt & Kuhnt, 1967), the parameters and configurations of the initial components of the VEP can no longer be distinguished from the VEP of the mature brain.

The only difference in the VEP to light between children and adolescents is the absence (or weak expression) and irregularity of the child's AD, which has also been noted in other studies (Cohn, 1964). As shown in Figure 4-6, this is registered with sufficient stability and a definitive latent period about age 14–15. At ages 6–8, 7–10-per-second AD bursts occur frequently, but later, for unknown reasons, their expression deteriorates sharply. Between the ages of 9 and 15, too, the third or fourth positive oscillation of the VEP is followed by the emergence of a slow negative wave 200–300 msec in duration, or by 2–3

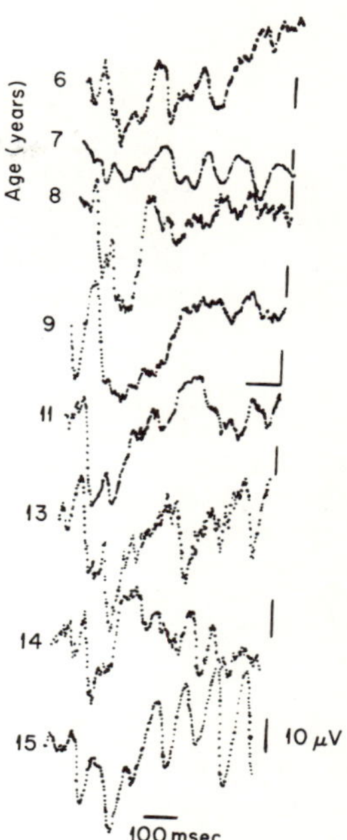

FIGURE 4-6. Individual VEPs in children of different age groups. (Numbers denote the age of the subjects in years.)

waves lasting 100–150 msec. If these are absent in the response to a single stimulus, they easily emerge in response to paired stimuli and greatly simplify the VEP configuration in children.

Metamorphosis of the VEP during Sleep. The general trends of changes in the EEG and VEP during sleep are shown in Figure 4-7. We have already encountered a similar reorganization of the VEP configuration. This suppression of the SAD and development of the SN occurred when light flashes were presented to a subject whose eyes were open or, more accurately, who looked at the light source. This transformation appears during the B stage of sleep (according to the staging of Davis, Davis, Harvey, & Hobart, 1938) immediately after the fourth positive wave, and less frequently after the third. This corresponds to a state of drowsiness, and the alpha rhythm is replaced by a flat high-frequency electric activity. Essentially, the SN appears against this same background during illumination with the eyes open. In any case it seems that the elimination of the alpha rhythm is required.

At the B stage of sleep, the SN is small; its duration does not exceed 70–100 msec. By the C stage (sleep of average depth), typified by the development of sleep spindles and individual bursts of theta waves, the amplitude and duration of the SN increase rapidly, reaching their maximum in the E stage of sleep (Figure 4-7).

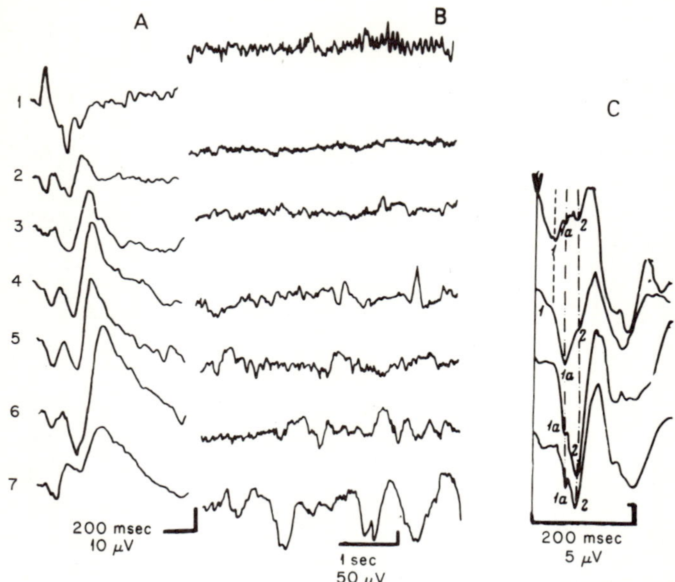

FIGURE 4-7. Visual evoked potential changes (A) corresponding to typical electroencephalographic stages of slow-wave sleep (B). 1, A stage of sleep; 2, B stage; 3, B–C stage; 4,5, C–D stage; 6, D stage; 7, E stage. Sleep staging according to Davis, Loomis, Harvey, and Hobart (1938). Some alterations in the EEG are due to sensory stimulation. Note the prominent slow negativity developing as slow-wave sleep progresses. C demonstrates short latency components of the evoked potentials in slow-wave sleep. It shows difficulties in description of metamorphosis of VEPs in a sleeping subject. The numbers *1* and *2* refer to waves P_1 and P_2; *1a* is an additional component not labeled in waking subjects. Here and in all subsequent figures tracings are the average of 20 responses. VEPs in A and in B are from different subjects.

In the C stage, the SN may be followed by a potential resembling the LR. Usually not more than 10–15 potentials should be averaged to bring this LR-type potential to the fore. It will be seen in the case of a consecutive, periodic averaging during the first two-thirds of stage C that there is a period when this potential is registered with sufficient constancy.

Finally, in paradoxical sleep the shape of the VEP very nearly coincides with that in stage B or the period of wakefulness. It seems that the VEP in the B stage of orthodox sleep differs only in a somewhat clearer expression of the SN whereas in paradoxical sleep there is a general flattening of activity following the P_4–N_4 complex. Thus, a clear picture of the qualitative changes of the VEP during sleep can be obtained and used for the purpose of classifying sleep stages. This yields somewhat different divisions from those determined by electroencephalographic studies.

The changes in the initial components of the VEP during slow sleep are also characteristic, even though more individual. The most constant changes are probably a decrease in the first positive oscillation (P_1) if it was visible in the period of wakefulness, and an increase in all other positive waves, especially P_2. However, in the case illustrated in Figure 4-7, there is an increase in oscillation P_1 (or to be more accurate, P_{1a}). The negative waves decreased, except for wave N_4 (or N_3), which evolved into the SN, and the generally very stable wave N_2.

Nevertheless, in some subjects more complex variants of evolution of the VEP during sleep were observed. The main difficulties in their evaluation resulted from the fusion of two neighboring positive components, which was caused by the reduction of the negative wave lying between them (generally N_1 or N_3). A case in point is the fusion of components P_1 and P_2, with which the VEP begins (see Figure 4-7). It is shown in the second VEP in that figure (the registration corresponds approximately to the C sleep period) that the P_1 component disappears and the positive component, which evolves from the additional wavelet of P_{1a}, becomes dominant. At this stage wave P_2 is seen only as a notch or deflection that can be traced on the descending slope of that new positivity. Later (the third VEP) there is an increase precisely in component P_2 and oscillation P_{1a} superimposes in the form of a variable peak on its ascending slope (D–E sleep). When sleep becomes somewhat less deep (last VEP on Figure 4-7) the amplitude of oscillation P_2 also decreases slightly and the separation of this summary positive wave into oscillations P_{1a} and P_2 becomes clearly evident. It will also be noticed that the growth of wave P_2 is attended by a simultaneous increase in the SN. Figure 4-7 shows a small section of its ascending slope.

Clearly, the most distinguishing feature in the reorganization of the VEP during the orthodox period of sleep is the emergence of the SN, which makes the human response resemble the VEP of a rabbit. If this is not a coincidence and the nature of the SN is identical in both cases, it can be assumed that the formation of W–S discharges is effected by the same mechanisms. This assumption has a number of implications—or, to be more specific, it presupposes a number of properties of the SN–LR of the human VEP.

We have only one indirect method of testing this assumption: analysis of the behavior of positive VEP waves, developing against the background of the SN. From the data given previously, we predicted the following properties to prove the similarity of the SN in man and rabbit:

1. Facilitation of the VEP positive waves will take place on the summit of the SN, when it just begins to decline (i.e., the development of potentials similar to A-potentials).
2. The time of facilitation will be inversely dependent on the sequence of its components. This means that, for example, the exaltation phase of component P_3 will take place prior to the intensification of wave P_2.

3. The dynamics of the curves marking restoration of the amplitudes of waves P_2 and P_3 must be identical during slow sleep and wakefulness with illumination directed on the open eyes.

These requirements should be satisfied if the positive components of the VEP of the human brain and the positive wave of the primary response in animals are of similar origin.

The VEP to a Paired Light Stimulus. Figure 4-8C demonstrates the evolution of the recovery cycle of the amplitude (A_2/A_1) of the more stable second and third positive VEP oscillations (P_2 and P_3). It can be seen that in the course of the restoration of these waves there is a basic exaltation period lasting about 100 msec, which is followed by a period of subnormality. It is better expressed in wave P_3; the amplitude of wave P_2 even decreases, although it still remains on a supranormal level. Then, as the interval between stimuli increases, there is a gradual increase in the amplitudes of both waves. After a delay of 300 msec, however, the second signal evokes the VEP, the amplitude of wave P_2 diminishes sharply, and P_3 continues to grow.

This picture of the restoration of the VEP is typical of waking subjects whose eyes are closed during light stimulation. There may be some variation in the time of emergence and the depth of the subnormality, the strength of expression of the initial rise in amplitude, and other characteristics. In this respect the data

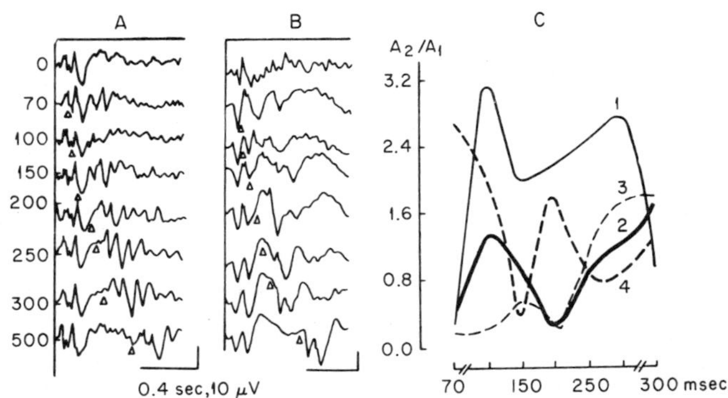

FIGURE 4-8. Averaged evoked potentials to double photic stimuli in A, waking state and B, in slow-wave sleep. Recovery curves in waking and sleeping subject are shown in C. A and B represent two different subjects. The first response in B was recorded in a waking state. Numbers on the left side of each trace in columns A and B indicate stimulus intervals between double stimuli in milliseconds. In C, the ordinate indicates amplitudes of P_2 (*1,3*) and P_3 (*2,4*) waves of evoked response to the second of a pair of flashes in a waking state (*1,2*) and slow-wave sleep (*3,4*). The abscissa indicates the interval between double stimuli in milliseconds.

given here confirm those obtained in other studies of the nature of the VEP recovery (Bergamasco, 1966; Schwartz & Shagass, 1964). However, it seems that the similarity in the dynamics of the restoration of the P_2 and P_3 oscillations, especially the coincidence in time of development of the first (and main) exaltation period, is not subject to variation.

We can now consider when the SN emerges and when and in what sequence intensification of the positive VEP waves occur during stimulation with the eyes open.

Figure 4-2 shows the dynamics of the recovery of the second and third positive VEP waves in three subjects in whom the similarity of the individual restoration curves appeared to be sufficiently significant. It is seen (Figure 4-2B) that with the subject's eyes closed the VEP oscillation recovery proceeds as just described. On the next graph (Figure 4-2C) it is evident that opening the eyes leads to a fundamental reorganization of the VEP restoration cycle. First, there is the exaltation of wave P_3; it is not noticeable when the second flash is delayed by 70 msec and reaches its maximum by 150 msec. Wave P_2, on the other hand, is not well expressed during the period of P_3 facilitation, and its intensification begins when the second stimulus is delayed by about 200–250 msec.

The same two periods of exaltation are observed when the SN appears during orthodox sleep: The early period develops at intervals of 70–100 msec, and the later period begins when the delay reaches 200 msec and more. As the interval between stimuli is increased, there is an intensification of the later positive waves P_4 and P_3 (early exaltation phase), followed by an intensification of the earlier P_2 component (see Figure 4-8B,C).

Thus, it can be concluded that VEPs in waking healthy subjects vary in general within rather narrow limits. When the variability of the VEP among human brains is mentioned, it is probably done to stress their individuality, which some authors compare with fingerprints. This individuality, noticeable despite the feebleness and extremely low amplitude of the response, is essentially the quality restricting its variability. It is likely that the perfection with which the brain masks its responses to afferent stimuli with the high level of "noise" caused by its spontaneous activity is an index of its health and stability. It is symptomatic that fluctuations in the direction of attention are generally not accompanied by serious changes in the VEP configuration. Changes in the form, the loss of individuality from a unification of the VEP, set in primarily with the advent of sleep, when the probability of the emergence of petit mal seizures is maximal (naturally, in people suffering from epilepsy).

The foregoing data give grounds to suspect that the SN is a result of two genetically homogeneous processes, which are therefore acting in the same direction. One of them is obvious in waking adults and is unmasked immediately with the blockade of the alpha rhythm.

The second process is connected with the slowing of background rhythmicity and the emergence of synchronized oscillations in the theta range, such as in childhood or during slow-wave sleep. In this case the SN increases in amplitude and duration in full accord with changes in background EEG oscillations. It may be assumed that the SN of VEP is similar to the SN of the cortical reaction to light in a rabbit. Both secondary VEP components seem to be related to the same process, i.e., sensory theta-rhythm of the occipital lobe. There is as yet no direct evidence, however, to show that the SN of the human VEP is but a "fragment" of the theta rhythm, and special studies are needed to test this assumption.

ABNORMALITIES OF VISUAL EVOKED POTENTIALS IN EPILEPSY

Electroencephalography came into its own after a successful debut in the clinics for epilepsy. Hence, great enthusiasm was evinced when the first attempts were made to study evoked potentials in epilepsy.

In 1947 Dawson showed that cortical reactions to stimulation of the peripheral nerves in epileptics were 5–10 times greater than in healthy persons. It was then thought that this was a discovery of universal significance. In any case there was no reason to believe that the VEP would prove an exception to what was almost regarded as a law. Soon, however, it appeared that paroxysmal facilitation of the VEP is only one of many possible directions for reactivity changes. New reports on the peculiarities of these changes in epilepsy seemed to increase exponentially.

Thus, a general increase in the VEP amplitude or a selective intensification of its various components was revealed (Broughton, Meier-Ewert, & Ebe, 1969; Cernacek & Ciganek, 1962; Ebe, Mikami, & Ito, 1963; Green, 1969; Weinmann, Heyde, & Creutzfeldt, 1966). There were also reports relating changes in the configuration of the VEP to the extensive increase in the amplitude and duration of the SAD (Bergamini & Bergamasco, 1967), or the development of the SN (Cohn, 1964; Morocutti, Sommer-Smith, & Creutzfeldt, 1966). Bergamini and Bergamasco (1967) also investigated the development of an SN in the VEP. However, unlike previous researchers, they only saw a long-lasting negative wave in some cases of centrencephalic epilepsy, and then in stage IV of slow sleep.

It would seem that the only consistent result was that the evoked activity of the brain in epileptics differs somehow from that in healthy persons. However, on this point, too, there is no unanimity (Hishikawa, Yamamoto, Furuya, Yamada, Miyazaki, & Kaneko, 1967; Lucking, 1969). The differences of opinion are so great that it is impossible to gain any clear idea about the direction of the changes in brain response, unless one assumes epilepsy is so multifaceted that the divergent effects result from the variability of the disease itself. Clearly, special research of the abnormalities of evoked reactions in epilepsy is more than justified.

I shall now describe evoked activity to light in patients suffering predominantly or exclusively from petit mal seizures.

Some Preliminary Remarks about the Cases Studied

General characteristics of the patients are given in Table 4-3. Most underwent at least initial clinical and laboratory examination in the Moscow Research Institute for Psychiatry of the Republican Ministry of Health. All patients showed classical absences, accompanied by 3-per-second W–S discharges. Some patients also displayed seizures of other types, such as grand mal (GM) or psychomotor attacks (PA). Late onset of the disease or the presence of a clear focus did not prevent inclusion in this group, if the absences themselves were clearly expressed and accompanied by the characteristic EEG pattern.

Electrophysiological studies were made prior to systematic treatment, or when possible, treatment was reduced during these studies. Twelve persons did not receive systematic treatment at all (in the drug response section of the table these cases are indicated by a question mark). In other cases the interruption of treatment was not dangerous because the patients were resistant to therapy (minus sign). Cases in which therapy was effective are marked with a plus sign; those showing considerable improvement, with two pluses; and complete control of seizures, with three pluses.

The column headed neurological findings shows the results of neurological and ophthalmological examination, X ray of the skull, and pneumoencephalography or arteriography. The plus sign is shown for cases in which the anamnesis indicates birth pathology, the presence of injuries of the skull, or contusion with loss of consciousness, even if the results of laboratory analysis were negative.

The EEG examination included visual analysis of the routine EEG, registration of the reaction to hyperventilation (duration 2–3 min), and study of brain sensitivity to flicker during wakefulness and sometimes during sleep. The EEG data given in the table relate to the background EEG in the interictal period. All patients could be placed in one of three groups in terms of electrical activity. The first group showed normal (N) EEGs, corresponding to age and without clear pathological signs. The second group showed episodic diffuse bilateral abnormalities (DA). These took the form of single or group waves in the theta–delta range with periodic bursts of W–S-type complexes, multiple spike–wave discharges, and the like. The last group included all cases in which, irrespective of the type of the abnormality, a stable asymmetry of its amplitude was observed. This was considered an indication of the presence of a focus (F). The corresponding section in the table indicates also the hemisphere (right or left) and the area (o, occipital; p, parietal; fr, frontal; t, temporal) in which focal

TABLE 4-3. Clinical Findings in Patients Suffering from Petit Mal

Case	Age (years)/sex	Age of onset of PM (years)	Neuro-logical findings[a]	History of other attacks[b]	Inducing factors	Routine EEG type/hemisphere–area[c]	Drug response[d]
K. L.	6/f	5			Flicker	N	+
M. M.	6/m	5	+		Flicker	F/L–fr	−
B. O.	8/m	4			Flicker, drowsiness	F/L–o	−
G. A.	11/m	11			?	N	−
O.	14/m	?			Flicker	F/L–fr	?
C. G.	15/f	?			Drowsiness	F/R–o	?
I. O.	15/f	6			?	N	?
L. R.	16/m	6	+		?	F/R–o	?
K. V.	17/f	8			TV, bright light	DA	++
S. V.	18/m	8		GM	?	DA	+
R. K.	18/f	?		GM	?	N	++
S. S.	18/f	10	+	GM	Drowsiness	DA	?
G. G.	20/m	17	+	GM	Flicker, fatigue	DA	?
K. J.	22/m	15	+	PA?	?	F/L–t	+
B. A.	22/m	9			?	F/R–o	−
U.	23/f	8			Flicker	N	?
S. N.	23/m	10		PA	?	F/L–t	−
A. M.	25/m	12		PA	?	F/L–t	?
Z.	26/m	14	+	GM	?	F(R>L)	?
G. M.	29/f	27?	+		Fatigue, drowsiness	F(L>R)	++

S. A.	29/m	18	+	GM	?	F(L>R)	+
T. N.	30/m	20	+	GM	Drowsiness	DA	−
K. K.	30/f	22	+	GM	?	?	?
L.	32/f	18?	+	GM	Street traffic, flicker, drowsiness	F/R—o,p	+
M. P.	33/m	25?			Emotions, fatigue	N	+
M. B.	34/m	15		GM	?	N	?
G. V.	35/m	26?	+	GM	Fatigue, drowsiness	DA	+
G-K, V.	38/m	24?	+	PA	Bright place, flicker	F/R—t, o	+++
G. A.	38/m	20	+	GM	Fatigue, drowsiness, flickering light	DA	?
R.	42/m	21	+	GM	?	F(L>R)	?
K. S.	43/f	?	+	PA?	Flicker	F(R>L)	−
P.	44/m	?			?	DA	−
G. S.	45/m	24	+	GM	?	F/R—o	−
T.	50/m	28	+	PA	Fatigue	F/L—t	−

[a]Plus sign indicates birth pathology, skull injury, or contusion with loss of consciousness.

[b]GM, grand mal; PA, psychomotor attacks.

[c]N, normal; DA, showing diffuse bilateral abnormalities; F, focus; R, L, right, left hemisphere; o, occipital; p, parietal; fr, frontal; t, temporal; > indicates direction of symmetry.

[d]Question mark, no systematic treatment; minus sign, patient resistant to therapy; plus sign, therapy effective; two pluses, considerable improvement; three pluses, complete control.

activity predominated. In a number of cases accurate localization of the focus was impossible, and only the direction of the asymmetry is indicated (L>R or R>L).

The VEP research included analysis of the reaction to a single stimulus in the visual and other brain areas, study of VEP dynamics to paired stimuli with varying interstimulus intervals (recovery cycle), and analysis of VEP evolution during sleep. The program required a minimum of 2–3 repeated studies, and in some cases studies were repeated 5–7 times with intervals of several weeks or months between them.

The statistical analysis in Table 4-4 gives the parameters of the VEP for a group of 25 patients, whose ages corresponded to those of a group of healthy subjects.

General Characteristics of Evoked Potentials to a Single Stimulus.   Two types of response were registered in epileptics. The form of one resembled the VEP of healthy subjects but the other was an abnormal configuration. Figure 4-9 shows the main variants of the VEP in epilepsy, registered in waking patients with their eyes closed.

The VEP of the first type is more widespread and was registered in 61% of all cases. Generally, if present, the AD is weakly expressed, although in some cases no abnormalities of the alpha rhythm could be found by visual analysis. In healthy persons, too, the AD may be absent, but in epilepsy its disorganization was more constant, similar to that registered when the eyes are open or during the initial stages of sleep. This may be related to lowering of alpha-rhythm stability and a longer depression in response to the stimulus. It should be borne

TABLE 4-4. Peak Latency and Amplitude of Components of Averaged VEP in Epileptic Patients (Mean ± Standard Error)[a]

VEP components	Peak latency (msec)	Amplitude (μV)
P_1	30.8 ± 2.20	6.1 ± 1.15
N_1	44.6 ± 1.13	7.1 ± 0.87
P_2	62.0 ± 1.80	14.5 ± 2.32*
N_2	98.7 ± 3.11*	13.5 ± 1.48
P_3	139.3 ± 3.30*	20.5 ± 3.39
N_3	178.2 ± 6.82*	15.9 ± 3.74
P_4	208.0 ± 6.45*	22.1 ± 4.13
N_4	247.2 ± 7.64*	23.3 ± 1.90

[a]All statistical analyses were performed on data of 25 subjects.
*$p < .001$.

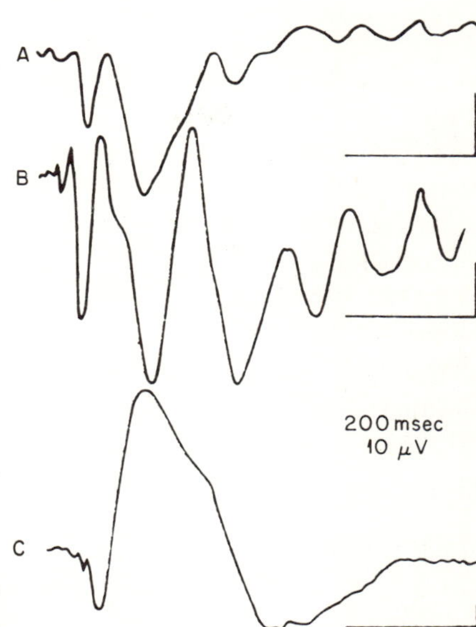

FIGURE 4-9. Examples of basic types of VEPs in patients having petit mal epilepsy.

in mind that the averaging of the VEP might be a factor in suppression of the AD, because of irregularities in the temporal characteristics of AD components.

Naturally, under these conditions even exalted waves of individual ADs will be suppressed, similar to the way in which random oscillations are eliminated. However, if the AD blockade is tied to the variability of its components, this does not preclude the disturbance of alpha-rhythm regulation in epilepsy.

In the response of the first type, which was related to the normal EEG classification, there is a clearly distinct N_4 wave (Figure 4-9A). In waking patients its amplitude and duration could attain magnitudes typical of the VEP during slow-wave sleep in healthy subjects (Figure 4-9A,B). The considerable predominance of the SN makes these VEPs resemble the W–S-type complex. Further, we shall refer to such VEPs as wave–spike reactions. It is interesting to note that when the patient opens his eyes or falls asleep the configuration of the wave–spike VEP does not change fundamentally (Figure 4-10). Perhaps normally this produces an unmasking of the SN, whereas in pathology the already unmasked SN is increased.

Wave–spike VEPs were registered in about 40% of all cases. However, we cannot consider this percentage stable since abnormal reactions to light could also appear in patients with an initially normal VEP configuration. Generally, this took place during or after light stimulation, especially in response to paired or rhythmical flashes; but a spontaneous VEP transformation could appear.

The amplitude of the wave–spike VEPs frequently exceeded the normal by two to three times or more, especially when such responses were registered in

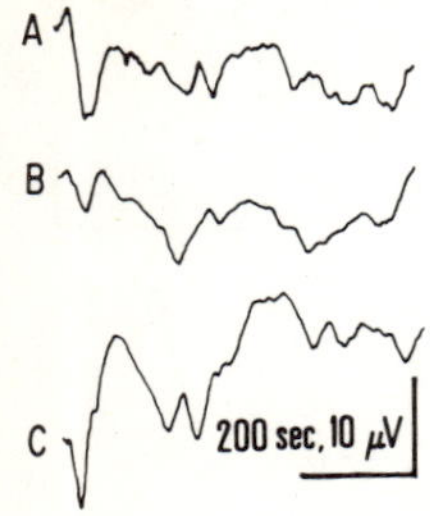

FIGURE 4-10. Minor changes in the secondary waves of the visual evoked potential in wakefulness and in slow-wave sleep in a patient: A, waking state, eyes closed; B, the same, eyes opened; C, slow-wave sleep.

children. This related to the cases demonstrated in Figure 4-9B and C. It would seem that wave–spike evolution of the VEP in children is generally explained by the clear expression of the slower VEP afteractivity at the early stages of ontogenesis, although such VEPs may be registered also in adult patients (Figure 4-10).

Table 4-4 shows the average magnitude of the VEP in a group of patients. It appears that an increase in the evoked reaction or its components should not be considered a universal symptom of brain epileptization. Wave P_2 is the exception, and it showed a statistically significant increase.

The VEP during Slow-Wave Sleep

In patients showing the stable normal type EEG, the VEP changes in brain reactivity during slow-wave sleep were virtually the same as in healthy subjects. The most interesting specific feature of the metamorphosis of the VEP during sleep in epilepsy was the appearance of a later VEP reaction (LR), following the SN. As in normal subjects, this occurred during the period of C stage when the K-complex was also clearly expressed (Figure 4-11).

It is reasonable that the configuration of the wave–spike VEP does not undergo other changes during slow-wave sleep (Figure 4-10). This suggests that the SN of waking epileptics shares an identity with the same component in sleeping normal subjects. Another implication is important for the evaluation of epileptiform EEG abnormalities. Since the SN of the rabbit VEP was shown to be derivative from the basic synchronous EEG rhythm, the same may be true for the human VEP, whether in sleeping healthy subjects or in waking patients. This implies that *slow-wave sleep EEG and hypersynchronous activity in epilepsy* could be phenomena of *similar* origin.

In REM sleep we have never seen wave–spike VEPs, though it is difficult to state that this is a consequence of active SN suppression and not spontaneous VEP normalization. Although the former is believed to be the case, as the SN is also suppressed during REM sleep in normal subjects, "spontaneous" VEP normalization was constantly observed in waking patients; I have stressed that wave–spike VEP is an unstable phenomenon.

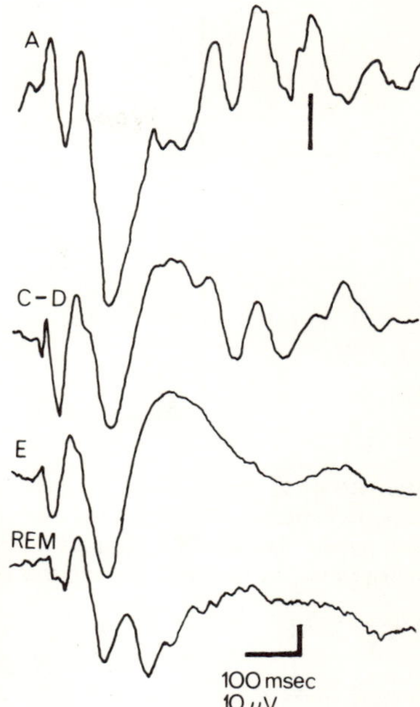

FIGURE 4-11. Changes in the normal-type VEP in an epileptic patient in different stages of sleep. Note a small deflection closing the SN and resembling an LR potential in C–D sleep and disappearance of the SN in REM sleep. Letters (A,C,D,E) refer to sleep stages according to Davis, Davis, Loomis, Harvey, and Hobart (1938) classification. REM represents rapid eye movement sleep.

VEP to Paired Light Stimuli.   Intensification of the VEP to paired stimuli was typical of most patients, irrespective of the VEP form. Sometimes the amplitude of the VEP components to the test stimulus exceeded that to the conditioning stimulus five times or more. In the presence of a wave–spike VEP a second stimulus evoked a second long-lasting negative oscillation in addition to the ordinary SN. Its maximum ranged from 400 to 500 msec, similar to the manner in which paired flashes evoke the emergence or an intensification of the AD in the normal brain. This repeated SN may also emerge in response to a single stimulus (Figure 3-9), but in the case of paired stimuli it was incomparably more stable. It is maximal for intervals between 100 and 200 msec and was present at practically all intervals studied.

It was found that the recovery cycle for P_2 and P_3 waves in epilepsy was very closely linked with the form of the VEP—or to be more accurate, with the presence or absence of the SN. The SN substantially changed the test response restoration process in a manner similar to that described for normal subjects in slow-wave sleep.

Figure 4-12B shows the restoration of P_2 and P_3 waves in a patient having an initial wave–spike form of VEP. It will be noted that if the VEP restoration is distinguished from that in normal sleep, it is due to more prominent test potentials in the exaltation phase. In another patient, the SN appeared during presentation of paired photic stimuli with an interval of 150–250 msec, and this

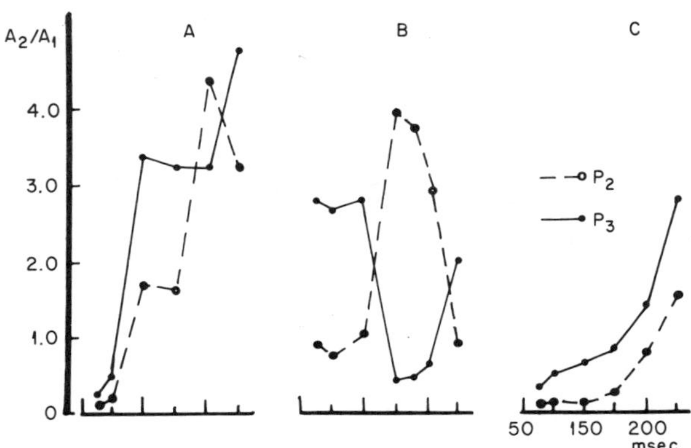

FIGURE 4-12. Comparison of the three basic types of excitability cycle of VEPs in epileptic patients. The ordinate indicates the amplitude of waves P_2 and P_3 to the second of two paired flashes. The abscissa shows the stimulus interval between double flashes in milliseconds. A, B, and C are recovery curves of different patients.

period marked the divergence of curves A_2/A_1 (Figure 4-12A). Increased sensitivity to flickering light was typical of both patients. In the first case the photoconvulsive reaction was provoked by a flicker at 11–15 Hz and in the second case, the flicker was 4–8 Hz, which can essentially be predicted from the properties of the restoration cycles. It is interesting to note that when wave–spike VEP developed, an increased photosensitivity to flicker presented with the eyes closed was observed. In other cases of photoepilepsy, it was preferable to activate W–S discharges in an eyes-open condition, when even healthy subjects show a hint of SN development.

Thus it might be that the substitution of the SN for the AD is a basis for the activation of the photogenic fit. In patients having photoepilepsy the SN amplitude was sometimes so pronounced that no averaging device was needed to separate the VEP from EEG "noise" to evaluate its type. Even when electrical activity was recorded with an ink-writing EEG machine, one could clearly see not only the initial wave–spike VEP, but also the low-frequency (3 per second) afterdischarge of a wave or wave–spike, resembling the AD in experimental animals (Figure 3-4).

The excitability cycles of the visual cortex described were not stable and were encountered along with normal forms in the same patient. The dynamic curve C (Figure 4-12) was more stable and was registered in one-third of the patients examined. It is interesting to note that one of them did not display increased sensitivity to flicker, although hyperventilation and/or falling asleep could activate paroxysmal activity.

PAROXYSMAL REACTIVITY OF THE BRAIN:
FRAGMENTS OF NON-REM SLEEP?

It has now been established that the amplitudes of the VEP as a whole or of its individual components do not essentially change in epilepsy. In this respect our data coincide with those of Hishikawa *et al.* (1967), Lucking (1969), Cernacek and Ciganek (1962), although the last probably observed a flattening of the VEP in epileptic patients. The controversy found in other studies is explained by lack of systematic observation, and also by inadequate estimations of the range of variability in normal reactions. Observations in healthy subjects showed that in some cases certain VEP oscillations were "excessively" increased. One has no choice but to interpret such an increase as a variant of the normal manifestation. Even when an increase in the VEP does take place in pathology, it is most frequently encountered in children, and is not a rule in other cases. This can be illustrated by the maximal amplitudes of individual VEP waves, which are rarely encountered normally. Thus, the magnitude, in microvolts, of wave N_1 was 17–20; wave P_2, 32–44; wave N_2, 28–40; wave P_3, 30–42; wave N_3, 45.8; wave P_4, 41–52.5; and wave N_4, 70. Although Green (1969) referred to similar magnitudes as "abnormally" increased, his data indicated that he had also found comparable values in healthy persons.

It is only partially true that the epileptic process leads to an increase and generalization of the early oscillations of the VEP to light (Broughton, Meier-Ewert, & Ebe, 1969). Wave P_1 may be increased, for example, but the possibility of its registration (as also of other VEP waves) in the rostral derivations is not a pathological symptom (Myslobodsky, 1970a, 1973). The significance of the dynamics of the VEP amplitude is still an open question, but in view of the ongoing controversy it is preferable for the present to turn to unambiguous symptoms, such as the asymmetry of the VEP or its relative changes at various stages of the disease. However, this question will be discussed in greater detail in the following section.

The most lucid reflection of abnormal reactivity of the epileptic brain was the change in the configuration of the VEP associated with blockade of the AD and the development of the SN. This was apparently also observed by other researchers (Morocutti *et al.*, 1966). It may be that such cases are more frequent than we were able to show in the present study, since the lability of the functional state of the brain in epilepsy is extremely high. In describing the reactivity of the healthy brain we paid attention to the great stability and individuality of its configurations. Although epilepsy does not erode the individual features of the VEP, there is a sort of unification of brain responses with the appearance of the SN and an extension of the range of their variability during the period of wakefulness. This VEP instability may be considered a characteristic symptom of the disease. It is comparable to the lability of the vegetative and metabolic processes in epilepsy (Sepp, Zuker, & Shmidt, 1947), which was vividly described as a "storm of fluctuations." This feature of the VEP may turn out to be a reliable nosological indicator.

The wave–spike evolution of the VEP also indicates diagnostic possibilities. The same is true of slowing the VEP beginning with wave N_2, apparently related to processes on which the formation of the SN is founded. However, abnormal VEPs were registered in various forms of epilepsy. In most cases they were encountered in persons with increased sensitivity to flickering light and the process of activation of a photogenic seizure sometimes closely resembled that encountered in animal experiments. But it is still too early to maintain that the appearance of the SN is simply a nosological feature.

Morocutti *et al.* (1966) observed VEPs of almost similar form during various kinds of epileptic syndromes. The illustrations given in the article by Broughton *et al.* (1969) indicate that wave–spike VEPs were registered in photogenic epilepsy as well as in the Unwerricht–Lundborg syndrome. The majority of researchers did not find abnormal configuration of the VEP in epilepsy. This was due to both an unsuccessful selection of patients and the short duration of analysis (up to 250 msec) of the brain responses (see, for example, Hishikawa *et al.,* 1967; Green, 1969; and others). It is also possible that the effectiveness of treatment differed, and this influenced the nature of the EEG and the VEP (Fridman, 1961).

At the same time the view that the SN appears only in centrencephalic epilepsy, and even then only during slow-wave sleep (Bergamini & Bergamasco, 1967) has not been confirmed. It was clearly expressed in all healthy subjects during that period. *The wave–spike evolution of the VEP is significant in epilepsy because it takes place during the period of wakefulness.*

Apparently there is no strict connection between the VEP pattern metamorphosis and definite forms of seizure. Classification of the disease on a clinical basis does not provide any key to the essence of epileptization, even in the group of minor forms. Yet they have something in common, something that unites the whole group of patients who have abnormal VEPs, irrespective of the nature of seizures.

The appearance of the SN coincides with the development in the EEG of pathological symptoms of a very definite category: slowing of the EEG, irregularity of the alpha rhythm, appearance of W–S discharges, separate theta waves, and groups of slow 3–4-per-second oscillations. Although the patients were awake, a situation developed that resembled the dissociation of the electrical activity of the brain and behavior in animals after the injection of atropine (Bradley, 1958). It appeared that the replacement of the sensory alpha-afterdischarge by the SN is an electrographic indicator of sluggishness, apathy, and inhibition, often signaling the proximity of a seizure. Thus, there are grounds to begin with neurophysiological and not clinical appraisal of data. To investigate pathogenetic therapy one must have data not only on the localization of the lesion of convulsive discharges, but also on the mechanisms or conditions that promote a pathological evolution of normal rhythmicity.

With most convulsive seizures one is justified in assuming that epileptic episodes of the grand mal type result from hyperdepolarization of the nervous tissue and its excessive excitation (Okujava, 1969), and that petit mal forms are related to an abnormal intensification of the feedback circuits. And if the former are accompanied by hyperactivity of the structures embraced by convulsive afterdischarges, the latter involve the inhibition of these structures. This interpretation mainly takes into account the nature of neocortical rhythmicity. Actually there may be considerably more complex correlations involving activation and/or inhibition of the subordinated systems, the spread of convulsive discharges, and a combination of the W–S-type complexes and convulsive afterdischarges at various levels of the brain, including the cortex. However, to simplify further discussion, we may say that these factors determine the specific clinical manifestation of the seizure. A more general, simplified scheme is acceptable since all variants of epileptic patterns may be reduced to the two polar types mentioned previously. Certain amendments to this scheme will be given here.

The most stable SN is registered in sick children. Hippocrates (cited according to Temkin, 1945) noted that epilepsy is a disease mainly of the young, and he considered its appearance after the age of 20 exceptional. According to Livingston, Torres, Pauli, and Rider (1965), in 93.1% of all cases petit mal emerges prior to the age of 13, usually between 4 and 8. It grows rarer with age, and if not complicated by grand mal seizures, may disappear without a trace. Hence, if there are normal rhythms and potentials that are transformed into paroxysmal ones, we should look for such forms and the conditions of their pathological evolution in children. It is therefore understandable that experimental petit mal seizures and W–S discharges, which are probably most closely related to human pathology, could only be produced in kittens up to the age of 1 month by the injection of aluminum cream into the rostral part of the brain stem, i.e., by stimulating the reticular formation (Guerrero-Figueroa *et al.*, 1963a).

It is commonly known that the EEGs of healthy children frequently show bursts of high-amplitude oscillations in the theta–delta range that resemble petit mal complexes. In infants and children the frequency of the basic rhythm ranges between 2 and 4 per second; in waking adults the emergence of such oscillations is undoubtedly considered a pathological sign. Fragments of mature rhythms may be registered in the same child, alternating with an immature, slow EEG picture. By 8–10 years of age a nearly definitive EEG is established, but in the beginning of the second decade of life, for unknown reasons, electrical activity again increases, and bursts or rhythmicity in the theta–delta frequency range are found. In adolescents, groups of waves at 2–4 per second with amplitudes of up to 60 μV, are registered very frequently in the occipital and parietal areas. They are of paroxysmal nature and may be mistakenly diagnosed as epileptiform (Farber, 1969; Gibbs & Gibbs, 1952). Correspondingly, in infants the VEP is distinguished by the presence of fully differentiated SNs or some slow negative oscillations resembling low-frequency afterdischarges (Farber, 1969). Naturally, in epileptic children these phenomena should be more regular, stable, and noticeable, and, as we saw, this is indeed the case.

There is a coincidence between periods of intensified synchronous electrocortical activity and greater probability of development of paroxysmal activity. This may lead one to conclude that the high degree of synchronization of the EEG is the pathophysiological basis of convulsive activity in children. Indeed, one frequently observes an intensification of oscillations in the theta range in the occipital areas of children suffering from petit mal seizures. Figure 4-13 shows that they are not only clearly expressed but are also asymmetrical. They are the most likely to evolve into W–S-type discharges during hyperventilation or presentation of flicker. At a higher flicker frequency that suppresses (desynchronizes) the rhythms, the probability of the development of a photogenic seizure is negligible. On the other hand, stimulation with paired or rhythmical stimuli at the same frequency as this rhythmicity leads to the appearance of a photogenic seizure. In other respects this is a fully normal rhythm, found also in normal children.

Obviously, hypersynchrony is the main, even if not the only, requisite condition for the formation of the SN. This is shown in experiments in which the SN is unmasked in normal persons when they are opening their eyes. I should add that it can also emerge from a breakdown of the mechanisms of alpha rhythmicity. In a number of cases these are parallel processes, and in some measure they determine the neurophysiological basis that unites pathological cases accompanied by reorganization of the configuration of evoked reactions. This, however, immediately raises a question about the mechanism of this change and about the nature of the SN as its most lucid indicator.

It may be that the clinical and EEG data for a large number of patients displaying wave–spike VEPs can be reduced to primary and secondary generalized forms in accordance with the terminology of Penfield and Jasper (1954). If we also accept the centrencephalic hypothesis of the genesis of epilepsy, then the SN must be regarded as a symptom of the activation of the nonspecific system. It would be a consequence of the intensification of the cortical reaction to a volley of impulses from the structures of the oral pole of the brain stem, which at that time are in a state of increased excitability. Since tradition links secondary VEP oscillations with the activity of these structures, this assumption seems fully warranted.

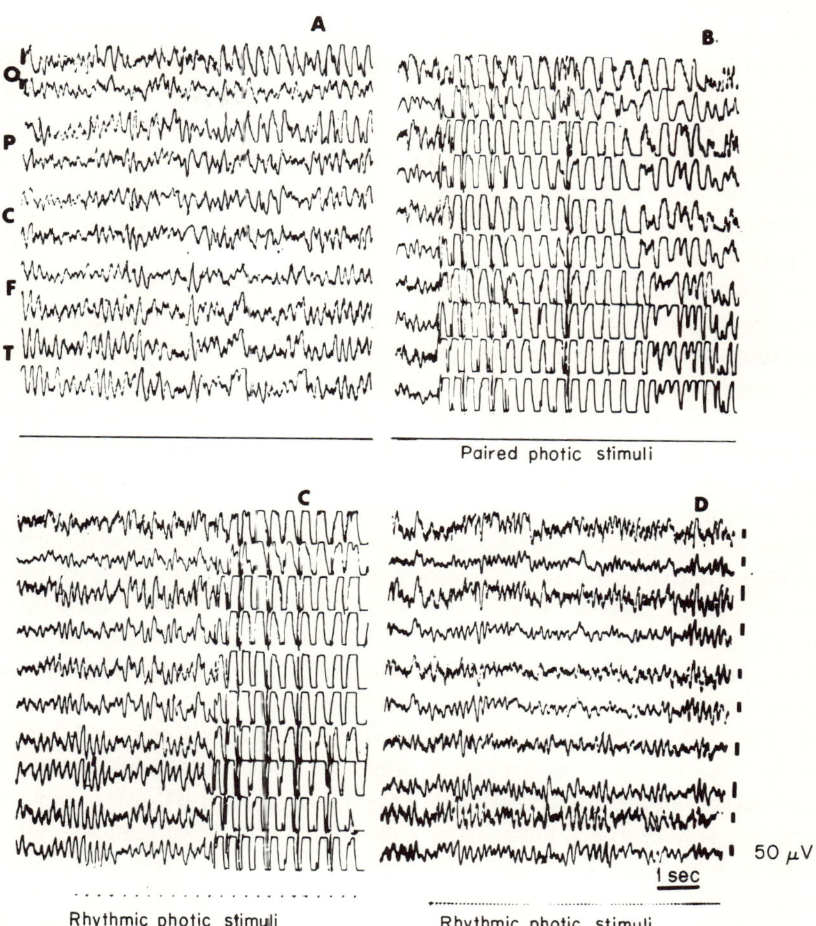

FIGURE 4-13. Bursts of slow posterior waves in a patient with petit mal epilepsy. A. Background EEG with posterior slow wave more pronounced in the left hemisphere. B,C. Photic activation of W–S activity associated with the potentiation of the slow posterior process. D. With the suppression of slow posterior rhythm (by high-frequency stimulation) it is impossible to activate the W–S pattern. Lower channel records the stimulus mark. Paired photic stimulation in B, and rhythmic in C,D. O,P,C,F,T indicate occipital, parietal, central, frontal, and temporal electrodes, correspondingly over the left (l) and right (r) hemisphere.

The foregoing is contradicted, however, by the great resemblance between the SN in man and the VEP in animals. The SN can emerge not only against the background of regular synchronized rhythmicity, but also against the background of a pathologically changed EEG. It is tempting to interpret this as "fragments" of sleep, as partial sleep of the cortex, which is compatible with the view previously outlined. If the synchronized sleep rhythm of humans is based on the same mechanism that phases depolarizing potentials with prolonged waves of postsynaptic hyperpolarization, then the SN may be one of the components of a multisynaptic but exclusively cortical process, which is triggered by an initial specific volley. It may also be that it is actuated by the activity of the mesodiencephalic centers only in the sense that their asthenia creates conditions for synchronous activity of the cortical cells and the organization of wave–spike VEPs.

This neurophysiological approach promotes an understanding of the wave–spike evolution of the VEP in the cases of lesions caused by tumor growth in the proximity of activating brain-stem centers (Melnitchuk, 1971). It also provides the sought-after common denominator for all pathological cases accompanied by changes in the VEP configuration.

The final appraisal of the causes of the readjustment of cortical reactivity in epilepsy will in many respects depend on what we are able to say about the nature of the components and, notably, the SN of the human VEP. The SN, obviously, is just as much a fragment of spontaneous rhythmicity as is the SAD, the only difference being that it is noticeable during the emergence of oscillations in the theta–delta range. That is why it is clearly expressed in childhood, non-REM sleep, and epilepsy. We register low-amplitude and irregular SNs in waking healthy subjects during light stimulation of the subject's open eyes and in the B stage of sleep, i.e., during the flattening of electrical activity. This shows that the mechanism on which the SN is based is to some extent the finale of the process triggered by a peripheral stimulus, and the SN is unmasked when the alpha rhythm is eliminated or when the physiological intensity of the stimulus is increased. This assumption may be viewed as a continuation of Lindsley's (1956) theory in which he drew a distinction between alpha rhythm and alpha activity for the other EEG frequency band. Thus, the SN is viewed as a reflection of a permanent theta–delta activity, which is the cellular excitability cycle phenomenon based on IPSP–EPSP sequences. It provides the other (i.e., apart from alpha activity) means for the selection and coding of afferent signals. When this process reaches its maximum it forms a distinct EEG rhythm of the corresponding frequency. This usually occurs with the lowering of cortical excitability. Thus, if we assume the existence of an independent extracortical source of inpulses evoking the SN, the reticular formation may perhaps be excluded as a possible generator, since its deactivation (or damage) leads, just the same, to a maximum increase of the SN.

We noted that the emergence of the SN makes the form of the VEP in humans resemble the cortical reaction in animals, although the situations in which this component attains its greatest expression are far less similar. This is probably explained by specific distinctions in rhythmicity; theta oscillations in rabbits, of which the SN is considered an evoked fragment, emerge in conditions of quiet wakefulness, when in humans the alpha rhythm is predominant. It would seem that the latter is a phylogenetically new mechanism, which might be seen as beginning in primates; and it is hardly worthwhile to compare it with the basic rhythm in the rabbit, as some researchers propose to do (Guselnicov & Supin, 1968). It would be more accurate to say that a breakdown of alpha returns the human brain to a phylogenetically more ancient level. However, the process of the VEP pattern transformation during changes in the background electrical activity greatly resembles that observed in rabbits. There in a state of wakefulness the SN—LR complex was the first component of the sensory afterdischarge (SAD). During narcotic sleep, however, the afterdischarge formed against fragments of barbituate spindles and the first stable component of the spindle was registered in the form of an "early" secondary response (Ivanitsky & Myslobodsky, 1965).

The similarity of the SN mechanisms is particularly striking when a comparison is made of the changes in the positive components of the test response developing against this SN background. When discussing the nature of the augmenting response, we arrived at the conclusion that A-potentials are related to the unmasking of the primary EPSP, against a background of postsynaptic hyperpolarization and its fusion with rebound depolarization. Since changes in the amplitudes of waves P_2 and P_3 against the background of the SN do not fundamentally differ from those found in animal experiments, we are justified in considering the SN of the human VEP to be a dipole reflection of the same EPSPs of the large pyramids that are generally masked by alpha rhythms.

If we make such an assumption with respect to the SN, we shall be compelled to extend it to the augmenting positive components. The similarity of their interaction with the SN implies a similarity between the genesis of the positive oscillations of the VEP in humans and the positive phase of the primary response in rabbits. I should add that light stimulation of the subject's open eyes also changes in the VEP characteristics in the predicted direction, decreasing the time to the maximum of oscillations N_1 through N_3 and slightly extending the peak latency to the wave N_4. Since the opening of the subject's eyes increases the physiological intensity of the stimulus, it may be assumed that the first components are predominantly depolarizing ones, and N_4 is mainly a hyperpolarizing wave. Thus, we are inclined to consider all oscillations of the VEP up to wave P_4 as analogs of the classical primary reaction (i.e., initial and later positivity), with the N_4 wave and the SAD as secondary potentials homologous to the SN in animals.

It is therefore very likely that this sequence of oscillations is an intracortical process, the development of which follows an initial depolarization process of specific origin. However, the same oscillations could also be evoked by the stimulation of some nonspecific inputs if the sequence of the VEP oscillations is also determined by a pacemaker or pacemakers in some subcortical centers. If we attribute this property to only one level of the brain, it must be proved that the cortical level is passive. The cortex of the animal brain is able to respond with primary and secondary reactions even in conditions of neural isolation; it would have to be shown that the cortical cells of the human brain have lost this property. We do not possess such data and I do not think that any will ever be found.

Thus, the existence of a sequence of heterogenous extracortical impulses each evoking a certain VEP component (Cigánek, 1961; see, however, Cigánek, 1967) seems doubtful. Like Creutzfeldt and Kuhnt (1967), we are inclined to relate the heterogeneity of the VEP in both human beings and animals to different degrees of participation in their organization by depolarizing and hyperpolarizing potentials, and not to differences in subcortical impulse sources. It may be added that in both animals and humans the primary and secondary VEP oscillations are specific reactions, the number, amplitude, and nature of which are determined by the logic of the activity in the excitatory and the inhibitory cortical circuits. Apparently the nonspecific limbic–reticular centers more or less selectively modulate the results of these specific activities at various points in the visual pathways. In view of this reasoning, it is believed that a certain similarity of the parameters and configurations of the VEP in normal slow-wave sleep and in epileptics is primarily due to the prominence of the inhibitory link in that circuit, because of an intensification of synchronous activity of the cortical cells. This phenomenon indicates also an infantilization of cerebral rhythmicity, which is expressed by its slowing and by an obscuring of the distinctions between sleep and wakefulness.

True, it is not impossible that the wave–spike VEP forms as a result of a more powerful initial afferent volley. However, in the event of synchrony of the geniculocortical volley there should be an increase in the amplitude and a decrease in the latency of at least some initial VEP oscillations, similar to the effect from opening the eyes. Only a significant increase in the amplitude of wave P_2 was observed in epilepsy; the time to the maximum of the initial VEP oscillations (including P_2) differed very little from normals. The time to the maximum of the other waves increased significantly, beginning with wave N_2. A slowing of the VEP was even noted when the pathological synchrony did not reach the level at which regular epileptiform discharges appear. Perhaps here light flashes exposed an endogenous propensity for synchronous response, but spontaneous hypersynchrony failed to manifest itself. The IPSP emerging in some elements is insufficient for the formation of the SN, but it is able to increase the latency of the VEP components.

In view of these discussions about the pathogenesis of petit mal epilepsy it would be premature to relate it exclusively to an abnormal intensification of postsynaptic inhibition. I emphasized earlier that excessively increased A-potentials were also registered in epileptic cases. Hence, it is essential to discover the nature of this additional process that turns an evoked potential in normal slow-wave sleep into a wave–spike VEP. Against this background augmented reactions become augmented paroxysmally and provoke a new A-potential–SN complex, i.e., a photoconvulsive reaction.

The analysis of the exaltation phase in the restoration cycle justified its being considered a combined process. It consists of excitatory postsynaptic potentials to the test stimulus fused with the depolarizing potentials of postanodal excitation, emerging after the end of inhibition from the preceding stimulus. This interpretation of the augmenting phase is of great importance for an understanding of the pathogenesis of petit mal forms of epilepsy, but the ideas must be considered from a somewhat different angle.

It was shown experimentally during single-unit recording in the visual cortex that the same VEP component—the so-called later response (LR)—always corresponds to rebound discharges. At the same time the SN of the VEP in the human brain only rarely ends with an LR. Normally the LR is registered exclusively during slow-wave sleep, and even then only during a rather short period in stage C. There is no certainty, however, that this episodic component and the LR that concludes the VEP of the visual cortex in the rabbit and rat are related phenomena.

In epileptic patients this component is sufficiently constant. It is more stable in non-REM sleep but in some patients it follows the SN of a wave–spike VEP during wakefulness. However, in this case, too, there is no certainty that the LR of wakefulness and sleep are related phenomena or that they are produced by the same mechanism that evoked identical VEP components in animals.

Hence, at first glance, it may appear that the process of reactivation of repeated W–S cycles is not identical with the similar phenomenon in rabbits, i.e., it is not linked with the mechanism of later (postanodal) discharges. However, one can proceed from the view that the exaltation phase is a combined event and that rebound depolarization participates in its organization. In this case the mere presence of an A-potential during the recovery cycle, especially in view of its excessive potentiation in epilepsy, is an indirect indication of the presence of mechanisms similar to those participating in the formation of the LR in the rabbit VEP. As I noted previously, in some patients suffering from photogenic epilepsy there is an intensification of the LR; and this, in full correspondence with theoretical predictions, leads to a reactivation of repeated W–S complexes of the photoconvulsive reaction.

The following amendments can thus be introduced into the considerations about the nature of changes in the reactivity of the cortex during petit mal forms of epilepsy. Obviously, in persons suffering from petit mal who have increased sensitivity to flicker, the activity of the excitatory circuits may be primarily damaged, too. It is not possible that they are circuits of recurrent activation. There are some data that indicate that the probability of additional appearance of grand mal is higher in this population.

ASYMMETRY OF HEMISPHERIC REACTIVITY IN NORMAL SUBJECTS AND IN EPILEPTIC PATIENTS

The Venetian Lancisi in the eighteenth century was probably the first who, when the "vital spirit" theory was still widely current, called the corpus callosum the *seat of thought.* This historical paradox is interesting only because quite recently the corpus callosum was reputed to be "the largest, most useless" structure (Sperry, 1962, p. 43).

At present, however, the idea is gaining ground (it has spread like an epidemic disease) that callosal fibers form the most important bridge between two "worlds," speaking different languages, distinguished by different ethics, logical systems, emotional levels, and modes of perception.

The link of the left hemisphere (in right-handed persons) with the functions of speech was recognized long ago (see Kok, 1967, for the literature). Its damage led to so serious a social defect that it has long since been named the *main, active, big,* or *dominant* brain. The voice and functions of the left were considered to represent the brain as a whole, and the overshadowed right hemisphere was therefore called *subdominant.* Quite recently new light has been thrown on the special, synthetic, generalizing functions of the subdominant hemisphere. In a review translated into English about 10 years ago, Lomov (1966) summarized some earlier studies on "bireception." He cited some data received in the early 1950s indicating the dominant role of the right hemisphere in weight perception, vibration, temperature sensitivity, and tactile discrimination. In a study conducted with Idelson (1966) the tactile recognition of different complex objects was estimated separately for the right and left hands in a group of right-handed subjects. Left-hand recognition was superior in 66% of the subjects. Right-hand superiority was found in 27%. In 7%, both hands performed equally. Later Nebes (1971) showed that the right hemisphere is able to determine the size of an object from incomplete information about it and to reconstrue the forms of fragmented figures. Defects of the right temporooccipital area (injuries, tumor growth, resection) led, correspondingly, to serious disorders of spatial thinking and analysis of visual images (Kok, 1967). Activation on the right hemisphere, for example that caused by irritative lesions, leads to visual illusions or the visual onset of an epileptic seizure (Penfield & Erickson, 1941). Human beings probably see dreams with the right hemisphere; in any case, their disappearance was described following the injury of the occipital lobes of the brain, affecting mainly the right hemisphere (Humphrey & Zangwill,

1951). Defects of the right hemisphere lead also to disturbances of musical ability (Kimura, 1964; Luria, 1970).

Even the functions represented in both hemispheres figure more diffusively in the right and locally in the left (Semmes, Weinstein, Gheht, & Teuber, 1960), which reflects the specific logic of the operation of the two brains. Lesions of the left hemisphere lead to a disturbance of concrete topographical perception, of orientation in spatial diagrams and maps; lesions of the right hemisphere lead to disturbances of orientation in real spatial situations (Traugott, Kaidanova, & Meerson, 1973).

Neurologists have long since encountered cases of depressive–catastrophical reactions in patients having defects of the dominant hemisphere (Gainotti, 1972; Penfield & Erickson, 1941), and reactions of indifference and euphoria, and anosognosia with defects of the subdominant brain (Gainotti, 1972; Kok, 1967). The cause of these astounding differences is as yet not quite clear. It may be related to different intellectualities of the hemispheres, which makes it possible to use the information theory of emotions to explain the phenomenon (Simonov, 1970). This theory relates emotion to the size of a deficit (negative emotion) or increment (positive emotion) in the requisite pragmatic information. Correspondingly, the more informed, intellectual, dominant hemisphere is more stable and has a reserve of positive emotions because of the definitiveness of the information with which it operates. The right hemisphere, on the contrary, works in a more generalized manner and has a chronic deficit of information, which according to Simonov's theory must be accompanied by negative emotional reactions. This explanation coincides with the views expressed by Hecaen and Angeleriques (1963), who also considered that the "primitivity" of the analysis of sensory information by the right hemisphere is the basis of its high-negative affective charge. However, this point of view does not explain why in a number of cases the hemispheres appear to demonstrate different affective polarities rather than simply varying intensity of affect.

Indeed, depressive reactions developed with pharmocological inactivation of the dominant hemisphere (homolateral intracarotid injection of Amytal), whereas the injection of an anesthetic into the right carotid induced a state of euphoria (Rossi & Rosadini, 1967; Terzian, 1964). It is very possible that peculiarities in the neurochemical organization of the hemispheres of the human brain might be responsible for these different reactions.

The ontogenesis of emotional reactions also suggests they are associated with different hemispheres. Negative emotions (weeping, sadness, disgust, anger, fear, and so on) are present practically at the moment of birth and seem to be definitely formed by the third month of postnatal life. Positive emotions (high spirits, positive excitement, attraction to peers and adults) begin to manifest themselves from the third month of postnatal life and form during the next 2 years in parallel with the development of speech (Tonkova-Yampolsky, 1971).

The left, "speech" hemisphere apparently operates according to the laws of formal logic, whereas the right hemisphere seems specialized for the analysis of images. The right hemisphere has in this sense a synthetic, generalizing function with respect to the more concrete dominant analytical mechanism (see Bogen & Bogen, 1969). In terms of Pavlovian physiology, in the right hemisphere sensory information is interpreted on the preverbal first-signal level; in the left it is generalized on the conceptual, second-signal level (Kok, 1967). Thus, we can conclude that the formation of the personality and the realization of the only goal of the brain—survival—are ensured by two fundamentally different systems, which (perhaps) have distinct structural and neurochemical foundations.

At a certain stage of research I did not take all this information into account. Electrophysiologists habitually carry out their experiments on one hemisphere, assuming that the data obtained apply equally to the other. True, in the experiments cited previously the activity of both hemispheres was virtually always registered, but this is in itself poor justification. These measures were motivated by a desire for "redundancy," with the intention of selecting the more successful of two reactions. Having two evoked potentials, I nevertheless always selected the VEP of the right hemisphere for processing. It generally seemed justified to analyze the reaction of the hemisphere "less subject" to external influences. One could give a number of reasons in defense of that viewpoint, beginning with the observation of the absence of a right hemisphere (discovered in postmortem examination) of some persons having normal intellect (O'Leary, 1967). In short, the VEP of the dominant hemisphere was shelved in expectation of better times and new ideas.

When studying the reactivity of the brain of epileptics, the maximally abnormal VEP or the VEP with the greatest amplitude was statistically processed, irrespective of the hemisphere from which it was recorded. The VEP of the other hemisphere was not taken into account at all. This naturally created certain inconveniences, and dissatisfaction was felt that the data were not really comparable. Some consolation was found in the fact that the VEP of the right hemisphere has a somewhat larger amplitude normally. By referencing to this deliberately exaggerated normative data we prevented exaggeration of the abnormalities in reactivity of the epileptic brain, which created a certain illusion of objectivity in the approach.

Soon, however, the situation became unbearable. First of all, when the forms of both VEPs were somewhat distorted, it was impossible to determine which of them was "more epileptic." Later it appeared that abnormalities in reactivity are not rigidly fixed and emerge now in the right, now in the left hemisphere in the same or repeated studies. Finally, statistical appraisal of abnormalities of reactivity was complex when they were compared with an abstract, averaged normative value, rather than with "their own control," i.e., the second hemisphere. It seemed that it was precisely here that the so-called individual abnormalities of reactivity, which could be related to differences in the reactivity of the hemispheres, were concealed. In short, all this prompted us not only to analyze archive materials (when possible), but also to appraise the dominance of the hemispheres in new cases of epilepsy. This was determined on the basis of questionnaires on "handedness," but since this criterion is only valid for right-handed persons, left-handed subjects were studied only in exceptional cases.

Let us, however, return to the problem of hemispheric dominance. The introductory information given here was essentially designed to demonstrate the mutual dominance of the hemispheres and to present some specific sphere of influence for the right hemisphere, which is in this connection described as *preverbal, synthetic, diffusive, prelogical,* and so on. This resembles a bustle of belated compliments to make up for the past neglect of this hemisphere. Most of us, however, live under the sign of the "social" left hemisphere, and in this sense it is more active, i.e., dominant. If this is so, the functional activity of the hemispheres must normally proceed at different energetic levels, which may be reflected in the differences of the hemispheric reactivity to a plain photic stimulus.

Reactivity of the Hemispheres of the Normal Brain

In 23 subjects (13 women and 10 men aged 18 to 37) the VEP was recorded to binocular photic stimulation, mainly in the eyes-closed state. The subjects were given no special instructions. A preliminary appraisal of the degree of the VEP asymmetry was made on the basis of a qualitative visual analysis. Statistical processing was used to determine the asymmetry coefficient of the amplitude and the VEP area. This coefficient (CA) was calculated as the amplitude or the area difference of certain components of the right and left VEP divided by their maximal value and expressed as a percent:

$$CA = A_r - A_l/A_{max} \times 100\%$$

where A is the amplitude or the area of a certain VEP deflection.

The first results in this series were disappointing. Group averaging, as well as individual results averaged from 30 or more potentials, revealed that asymmetry of reactivity to a plain photic stimulus was only marginal in about one-third of the subjects and was not visible at all in others.

However, when a smaller number of potentials was averaged it became clear that interhemispheric VEP asymmetry does exist. A brief methodological digression should be made before these results are presented.

In epileptic patients photic stimulation was preferably presented in periods when EEG abnormalities appeared or grew more visible. This is a natural diagnostic approach, similar to that used with conventional EEGs. It allows recording of wave–spike VEPs that would otherwise remain unclear. Averaging potentials across different EEG backgrounds could provide information on the general state of brain reactivity during certain periods of time. However, averaging the VEPs from varying backgrounds makes neurophysiological evaluation of the data problematic. Associating stimulation with a particular EEG background is an important requirement if one does not expect dramatic VEP changes, as in studies of VEP asymmetry.

The reactivity of the cortical circuits is conceived as a cyclical process. For practical purposes it is preferable to limit oneself to two main cycles, which if unrestrained are able to affect the final VEP parameters. One cycle corresponds to alpha-spindling periodicity, whereas the other coincides with intraspindle excitability changes (Andersen & Andersson, 1968). By presenting the photic stimuli on brief fragments of the desynchronized EEG between spindles, one is able to avoid interference with the cyclic changes of the alpha-rhythm excitability. The signal operates during a more desynchronized period, corresponding to the period of alpha process (Lindsley, 1956). Thus stimulation against the background of alpha spindle, which requires the presentation of the stimulus on certain portions of the alpha waves, was avoided; not more than 20–25 stimuli were averaged in one stimulation session. Each session was repeated five times and the degree of VEP asymmetry was evaluated on the basis of five separate VEPs.

Even with this approach, nearly symmetrical primary components of the VEP were recorded in all subjects. However, in 18 subjects at least three out of five VEPs had a higher AD amplitude over the subdominant hemisphere. In 7 subjects this AD asymmetry reached 20–25% and was statistically significant ($p < .05$). It was eliminated when stimulation was presented in an eyes-open state (Figure 4-14) despite a somewhat higher AD amplitude remaining in the right hemisphere.

Thus, the hemispheres react in different ways to a simple light signal. It is noteworthy that it is not the whole VEP that changes, but only a certain component of the VEP, and this may receive a rather traditional, straightforward explanation.

It is known that reactivity is asymmetrical during presentation of stimuli that specifically activate the functions of one hemisphere or the other. When this is done the VEP to specific signals increases. Thus visual presentation of a word signal causes an increase in the evoked potential of the left hemisphere (Buchbaum & Fedio, 1970). Presentation of a speech stimulus, as distinct from simple clicks, evokes an intensified potential in the left temporal parietal areas (Morrell & Salamy, 1971). Admittedly, there are some who would argue against this simple conclusion. The visually presented word is a specific signal for the left hemisphere since it is a verbal stimulus; the same word, however, is perceived as

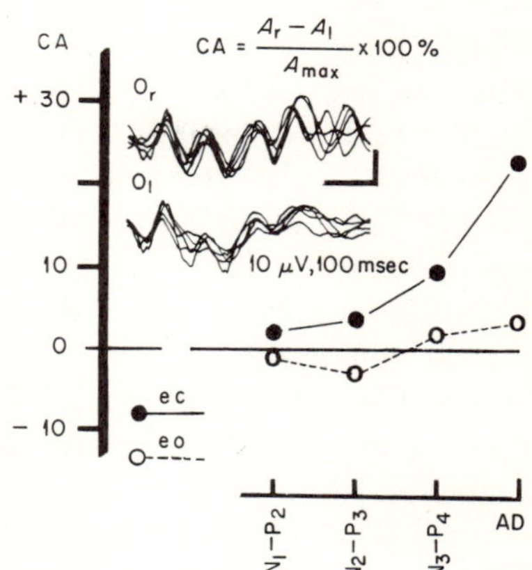

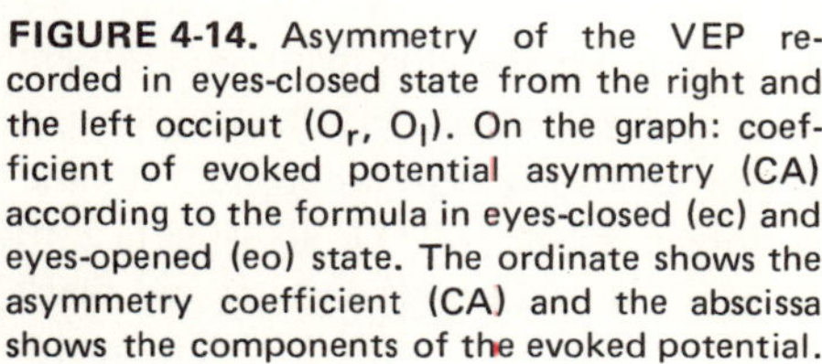

FIGURE 4-14. Asymmetry of the VEP recorded in eyes-closed state from the right and the left occiput (O_r, O_l). On the graph: coefficient of evoked potential asymmetry (CA) according to the formula in eyes-closed (ec) and eyes-opened (eo) state. The ordinate shows the asymmetry coefficient (CA) and the abscissa shows the components of the evoked potential.

a geometrical pattern and thus is equally specific for the right. Indeed, Shelburne (1972) did not corroborate the data submitted by Buchbaum and Fedio (1970). During isolated stimulation of one hemisphere (monocular stimulation of the right or left visual fields) by a simple light stimulus, Vella, Butler, and Glass (1972) did not discover VEP asymmetry. However, when stimulating with a complex checkerboard signal they received an intensified response in the right temporal derivation, due mainly to a component apparently corresponding to wave P_4. This effect was noticed during stimulation of both visual fields, but a particularly substantial facilitation of the VEP took place during stimulation of the right hemisphere through the commissural pathways, when a facilitation was recorded even in the occipital derivations.

The first systematic research on the asymmetry of hemispheric reactivity, undertaken in Beck's laboratory, was made with ordinary binocular stimulation using a plain photic stimulus. It appeared that in normal waking subjects the VEP amplitude predominated in the right hemisphere, especially in the central derivations. It disappeared following the consumption of alcohol (Lewis, Dustman, & Beck, 1970), and it has not been found in newborns (Groth, Weled, & Batkin, 1970) or mentally retarded children (Bigum, Dustman, & Beck, 1970; Rhodes, Dustman, & Beck, 1969). This suggests that the asymmetry of the reactivity of the brain hemispheres is a necessary condition for its normal activity. However, in these studies, asymmetrical intensification of the VEP components preceding the AD was constantly seen.

In 1964 Cohn discovered an intensification of the AD of the VEP in occipital derivations of the subdominant hemisphere. This observation, however, was subjected to question in later studies (Peacock, 1970). In the conditions of the present study, asymmetrical SAD was the exception rather than the rule as far as the tendency is concerned. It is likely that this effect has a natural explanation, since the AD is an evoked variant of the alpha rhythm.

Intensification of the alpha rhythm in the right hemisphere attracted the attention of researchers at the dawn of the development of electroencephalography. It is first mentioned, as far as we know, in the writings of Cornill and Gastaut (1947), who observed alpha asymmetry in normal waking subjects in 58% of all cases, which is somewhat higher than the AD asymmetry percentage found in this study. Later this result was substantiated in a number of studies. It was also shown in these studies that during mathematical and verbal operations the alpha-rhythm blockade is more noticeable in the dominant hemisphere (Butler & Glass, 1974; Morgan, McDonald, & MacDonald, 1971). Also, during visual imaging a relative lowering of the alpha-rhythm amplitude in the subdominant hemisphere is observed (Morgan *et al.*, 1971). Idelson (1966) demonstrated asymmetric changes of the EEG in subjects during isolated work with each hand. When a subject manipulated an object with the right hand, contralateral EEG changes were primarily seen. For left-hand activities, bilateral EEG suppression was observed.

Researchers display a rare unanimity toward the alpha rhythm. It has been regarded as an indicator of rest, relaxation, and lowered attention—in short, as an inhibitory brain state. Hence, the relative predominance of the AD on the right may be a symptom indicating that the subdominant hemisphere operates in a somewhat inhibited state.

Although it was difficult to doubt the existence of AD asymmetry, it remained to be found why it is so unstable. Figure 4-15 summarizes VEP changes under the influence of "selective" activation of the hemispheric functions. The subjects were instructed to execute operations with words or mathematical computations on command. These included finding a word to rhyme with a given word, finding words containing a given number of letters, multiplying, finding the square root of various numbers, and so on. Another instruction required the subjects to think of some concrete image or picture while trying to avoid verbal associations. After preliminary experiments all subjects preferred an approximately identical set of images: pictures of a ruffled sea periodically reflecting sunspots; clouds traveling in the sky, episodically revealing the sun; the shaking of the crowns of trees on a clear, windy day; and other pictures that included light stimulation as a factor changing the illumination of the image. This element was included even if a subject preferred concrete images (the face of mother, girlfriend, etc.).

Despite accurate evaluation of the difficulties and attempts to concentrate on a preferred image, only three subjects maintained that they were able to hold on to the visual image during stimulation. The others stated definitely that this task was beyond their powers. It is interesting to note that when the subjects were solving problems or imaging the amplitude of the background EEG decreased, irrespective of the nature of the task. However, during imagery tasks the EEG amplitude showed a greater decrease. The involvement of both hemi-

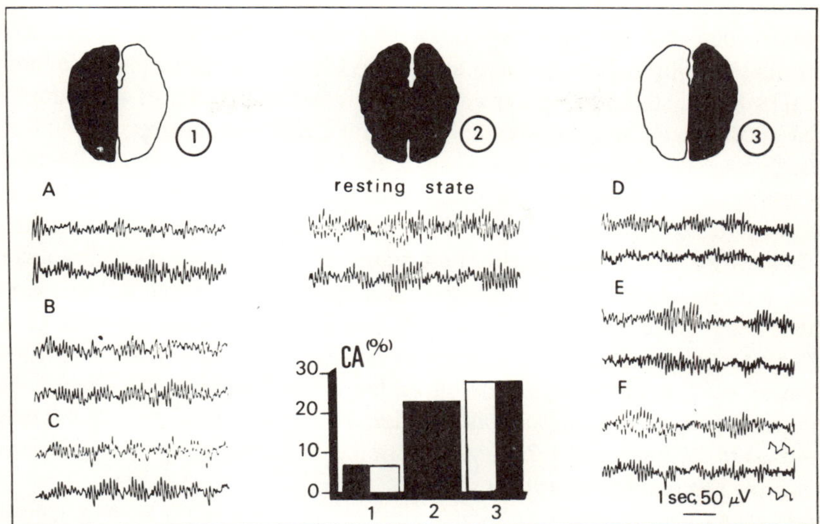

FIGURE 4-15. Interhemispheric relations of the EEG and visual evoked responses during (1,A-C) visual spatial test, (3,D-E) analytical test, and (2) resting state. EEG samples were taken during photic stimulation while subject relaxed (2, resting state), tried to imaginatively picture a storm at sea (A), floating clouds (B), mother's face (C), or to solve bourime problem (D), recall words with a specified number of letters (E), or multiply numbers (F). Upper traces are from the right hemisphere; lower from the left. The graph shows the dependence of the asymmetry coefficient (CA) for the secondary part of the visual evoked potential (P_4—alpha afterdischarge) amplitude on the task content. 1. Visual—special task. 2. Resting state (relaxed wakefulness). 3. Verbal—numerical (analytical) task.

spheres in an analysis of the specific task was noted as early as 1940 by Lindsley; however, in some cases specialized activation of one of the hemispheres, reflected in the selective decrease of the alpha-rhythm amplitude, is still sufficiently noticeable (Figure 4-15). A study of the amplitude from the peak of wave P_4 to the maximum of the negative AD of the VEP is more illustrative in this sense. The amplitude of these components decreased significantly on the left during the solution of mathematical problems and operations with words ($p <$ .05). When carrying out imagery tasks the decrease of the P_4–SAD amplitude was noted predominantly on the right. However, this result was statistically significant in only one subject.

Interrelation of VEPs of the Hemispheres during Sleep

The functional asymmetry of the human brain has been inferred exclusively from studies conducted in the waking state. It may be questioned whether the model of hemispheric asymmetry is valid for sleep, with its peculiar type of mental activity, dissimilar perception, and decreased ability to learn new material or respond to stimuli.

When a person is falling asleep a radical change of the VEP configurations takes place in both hemispheres, and the VEP pattern is identical in both hemispheres. A statistical analysis demonstrated that differences between the VEPs of the right and left hemispheres during sleep are greater than during wakefulness. The asymmetry coefficient of the SN area was calculated. The SAD area served as a reference for the comparison of VEP asymmetry in the waking state with that in sleep. In Figure 4-16, the dynamics of the SN asymmetry coefficient are plotted across different states of sleep. The figure shows that during wakefulness (or stage O) the asymmetry coefficient of the AD area has a positive sign (predominance of the AD on the right). With the advent of slow-wave sleep, the sign of the asymmetry coefficient changes (relative predominance of the amplitude and duration of the SN in the left hemisphere). This asymmetry persists with episodic fluctuation during 4–5 hr of sleep and it may be preserved for the first 10–20 min after awakening, even though the VEP form has returned to that of the waking state.

The broken lines of Figure 4–16 indicate the results during the second night in the same subject. Rather satisfactory coincidence with the first night is evident. The same reversal of the asymmetry coefficient was revealed in all four subjects studied in this series, although in others the periodicity of the changes of the coefficient sign was different.

Unstable or suppressed secondary VEP components made it impossible to study the hemispheric reactivity during REM sleep. Nevertheless the impression was gained that primary VEP components are practically symmetrical during REM sleep.

Let me now give a brief summary of our findings in this section. In normal waking subjects the AD of the right hemisphere VEP may be 25% higher than that of the left. This may be related to the lesser activity of the subdominant

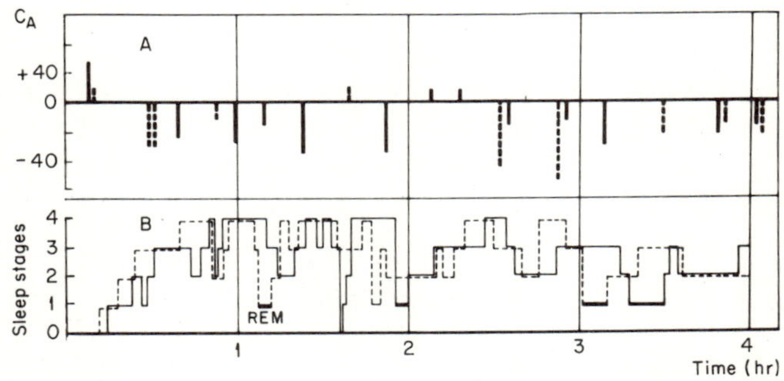

FIGURE 4-16. Changes of the coefficients of VEP asymmetry (CA) (asymmetry of the area of the AD and the SN of the VEP) in normal subjects during sleep. In A, the dynamics of CA are indicated by columns corresponding to different stages of sleep shown in B. Solid columns and lines indicate the first night. Broken columns and lines indicate the second night, same subject.

hemisphere. This is also expressed by the degree of complexity of the spontane-ous organization of a visual image and the subject's difficulty in retaining that image, be it a geometric figure or complex picture. It would seem that at a mature age eidetic abilities are a rarity, and the preference for using the left dominant hemisphere for the solution of regular problems becomes a sort of neurophysiological mechanism. In this sense it might be as well to continue calling the left hemisphere dominant. However, the language hemisphere is not always dominant or more active in this sense; sometimes in right-handed individ-uals a more prominent AD is seen in the left hemisphere. We have seen only three such persons, but the finding itself was rather stable from trial to trial. In those cases the solution of verbal and mathematical problems lead to the obvious supression of the AD as in other subjects, imagery tasks evoked for the most part bilateral suppression of afteractivity.

It is certainly difficult to evaluate these findings properly now; even so, I am ready to assume that the very fact of predominance of the AD in the left hemisphere points to its having lower activity in some right-handed subjects. This suggests that dominance is some common denominator of the personality, an indicator of how perception and thinking proceed. They may follow the "image" type comprehension typical of children and persons with an "artistic" makeup according to the definition of Pavlovian neurophysiology, or they may be based on the logical "sectioning" of data, with abstractions and generaliza-tions and verbal designations, typical mainly of persons with an "intellectual" makeup.

In the previously cited paper of Butler and Glass (1974), which appeared after our preliminary data had been published (Myslobodsky, 1973), we found an interesting explanation of the controversy between researchers who found alpha asymmetry in the EEG and those who did not. Butler and Glass suggested that EEG asymmetry may be associated with an analysis of the situation, which the subject makes inadvertently when he is exposed to the recording procedure.

In our study the subject was always positioned in a soundproof room. However, the assumption of Butler and Glass caused us some apprehension, and after reviewing our study, I found that six subjects with predominant right-sided AD had known the theoretical objectives of the experiment and had participated in their discussion. They were students and colleagues; and in this sense the initial AD asymmetry in this experiment may be an artifact, resulting from the subject's analysis of the situation and his expectation and prediction of its results. Even if it is an artifact, it is one that confirms rather than contradicts the final conclusion of the experiment.

Finally, the study of sleep showed that the amplitude and duration of the SN during most of the period of slow-wave sleep is greater on the left. If the assumption is correct that this component is an integral indicator of the depth of orthodox sleep, it is also correct that the inhibitory processes in the right hemisphere are less intense in slow-wave sleep than in the left. This means that the relative predominance of activity in slow-wave sleep tends to favor the subdominant hemisphere. In other words, there is a day—night interchange of dominance when the *wakefulness-dominant* left hemisphere becomes *sleep-subdominant*. Thus the question of which hemisphere should be considered dominant may be meaningless, unless the period is specified during which such domination applies.

The negative affective charge of the right hemisphere gives reason to speculate that the predominance of its activity in sleep may be the source of arousals with highly aversive mentation, such as night terrors. These do arise out of slow-wave sleep, and it is during slow-wave sleep that the vigorous electrodermal activity, so-called "GSR storms," were described (Broughton, Poire, & Tassinari, 1965).

Reactivity of the Brain Hemispheres in Epilepsy

Twenty-two right-handed patients were selected for this analysis. Information on them is given in Table 4-5. The asymmetry coefficients of the amplitude and the area of the secondary VEP components (P_4—AD and derivative abnormal complexes like the SN) were computed for all patients. Hemispheric differences of the primary VEP deflections were not taken into consideration because of the enormous number of variants.

The data obtained made it possible to divide patients into three main groups:

1. Those with symmetrical VEPs (asymmetry did not exceed 25%). This group of patients showed the normal type and wave—spike VEP patterns. Some of them had clear focal abnormalities in the rostral leads.
2. The second group consisted of only two patients, who had stationary VEP asymmetry. Both displayed clear focal abnormalities (in the temporal area in one case and in the parietal in the other).
3. This group included patients with normal and abnormal VEP patterns, but with asymmetry exceeding 25%. Unlike the previous group, asymmetry was unstable. Even during a single recording session the VEP could normalize or increase in amplitude and assume a somewhat distorted shape, while in the other hemisphere the VEP potential might be normal.

All these cases were selected for VEP analysis during a certain period on the basis of EEG abnormalities revealing identical dynamics. Hence, the actual number of population with such an unstable type of abnormality is unclear.

Although such asymmetry was called *dynamic,* it was actually due to some abnormalities in the right hemisphere. Indeed, if the asymmetry coefficients obtained from different recording sessions were arranged according to the magnitude of their positive values and the maximal figures for the reversed

TABLE 4-5. Clinical Findings in Patients[a]

Case	Age (years)/sex	Age of onset of PM (years)	Neuro-logical findings	History of other attacks	Inducing factors	Routine EEG type/hemisphere —area
S. P.	7/m	4	+		?	F/R—t, fr
K. K.	9/m	8			TV	N
L. O.	9/f	9		PA?	?	N
I. P.	10/m	5			Flicker	N
K.	11/m	6		GM	Drowsiness	N
G. N.	11/f	?	+		Flicker	F/R—fr
S. N.	11/m	4			Flicker	N
R. I.	12/m	8			Bright light	N
R. U.	13/m	8	+	PA	?	F/L—t
N. Ju.	13/f	6		GM	?	N
C. Z.	13/m	10		GM	Drowsiness	DA
S. V.	16/m	9		PA?	?	F/R—fr
P. K.	16/f	?	+	PA?	?	DA
E. A.	17/f	13			Flicker	DA
L. G.	18/m	10	+		?	DA
V. P.	18/m	9		GM	?	N
C. Z.	18/m	7			?	N
L. K.	18/m	?			?	N
A. L.	20/m	16	+	GM	?	DA
M. A.	22/f	11	+	GM	?	DA
A. G.	23/m	8		PA, GM	Drowsiness	F/L—fr
V. K.	23/m	16	+	GM	Fatigue	DA

[a]See Table 4-3 for an explanation of symbols used.

asymmetry coefficients were plotted simultaneously, as shown in Figure 4-17A, the VEP amplitude of the left hemisphere predominated in only 3 patients out of 10. The graph shows that an increase in the positive values of the asymmetry coefficient in some patients was not accompanied by a simultaneous increase in its negative values. On the contrary, the increase in the positive values of the asymmetry coefficient was accompanied by a lowering of the negative one. Only in two cases was there a true reversal in the sign of the asymmetry coefficient; in all other cases the magnitude of the coefficient did not even reach the value fixed as a criterion for normal asymmetry for secondary VEP components.

Correspondingly, in 6 patients out of 10 the occurrence of right-side VEP predominance was more probable; in one case right and left predominance of the

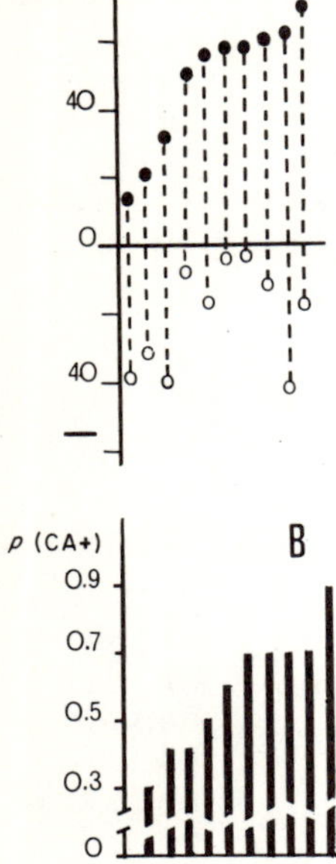

FIGURE 4-17. Asymmetry coefficient of visual evoked potentials in epileptic patients with dynamic asymmetry of brain reactivity. Each vertical column in A indicates maximal value and the sign of the factor in each patient. B shows probabilities (p) of positive values of the factor in the same patient.

VEP was encountered equally frequently; and in three cases the left-sided VEP increased (Figure 4-17B).

The normalization and reversal of the asymmetry coefficient stems from changes in the reactivity of both hemispheres. When positive asymmetry coefficients are changed to negative ones, this is accompanied by a decrease of the VEP amplitude of the right hemisphere (by 60–65%) and a simultaneous increase of the VEP in the left hemisphere (about 50%). At that time the VEP of both the right and the left hemispheres may decrease somewhat.

Thus, at least 50% of the patients having petit mal seizures display a stationary or dynamic VEP asymmetry. Stable VEP asymmetry coincided with the orientation of the focus; however, "symmetrical" VEPs were also registered in cases where there was clearly a focus. Evidently, occipital VEP cannot serve as an integral indicator of pathology if the focus is remote from the recording electrodes.

The existence of focal lesions outside the centrencephalic system in petit mal epilepsy is not a new discovery and has long been used in the polemic against the centrencephalic theory (see Chapter 1). Focal discharges of the W–S type are also known to be rather frequent events. It would seem that the focal VEP transformation into the wave–spike type found in this research is associated by the corresponding development of slow focal rhythmicity. These asymmetrical wave–spike VEPs do not differ from symmetrical wave–spike VEPs in normal people during sleep or in epileptics with symmetrical responses. Perhaps the mechanisms of the reorganization of cortical reactivity in all the cases mentioned are related. The difference is, apparently, that symmetrical wave—spike VEPs are evoked by some common cause leading to disturbance of the control of cortical rhythm in both hemispheres, whereas local wave—spike VEPs result from a limited disturbance in the executive mechanisms by which subcortical afferents controlling cortical rhythmicity are operated. The common features of local and bisynchronous wave—spike VEPs makes one suspect that they are associated with some mechanism causing the deafferentation of the cortex (local or generalized), and not with the influences of some specialized inhibitory pacemaker center. If the dynamics of the activity of the epileptic focus are compared with the evolution of brain reactivity in sleep, it must be admitted that the same transitional VEP forms may also be typical of a local cortical epileptic lesion.

Another interesting finding was the dynamic VEP asymmetry together with a higher probability of intensification of the secondary VEP components in the right (subdominant) hemisphere. This logically provokes the question whether this should be regarded as a sign of higher vulnerability of the subdominant hemisphere in petit mal epilepsy.

Lesions are encountered more frequently in the left, not the right hemisphere, especially for temporal lobe epilepsy. To explain this puzzling phenomenon Taylor and Ounsted (1971) suggested an interesting hypothesis. It is based on ideas about the heterochronous development of the hemispheres and, hence, their differential vulnerability at early stages of ontogenesis (see Chapter 2). It is assumed that the left hemisphere matures later than the right, and, correspondingly, runs a greater risk of being damaged by generalized cerebral pathology of any origin. The critical period for the right hemisphere is apparently the end of the prenatal and the first months of the postnatal period. In any case, prenatal injury leads to the development primarily of right-side lesions; postnatal injury leads primarily to left-side lesions (Zemskaya, 1971). This hypothesis helps explain the lateralization of the lesion during later onset of epilepsy, proceeding from the widespread pathophysiological principle that a stress-provoking agent initially decompensates the hemisphere damaged during the early stages of ontogenesis.

This principle is also applicable to petit mal epilepsy, which has already lost its distinction as an "elite" cryptogenic pathology, supposedly not linked with any organic defect of the brain. Abnormalities may be found in patients suffering from absences, testifying to prenatal and postnatal brain damage (Holowach, Thunston, & O'Leary, 1962) and leading to a decrease in IQ (Charlton & Yahr, 1967).

This hypothesis, however, does not explain the particular case of asymmetry of electrical activity of the brain that is unstable and may be described as a "dynamic focus." Such migrating lesions have been observed by many researchers (Gloor, 1972; Hess, Scollo-Lavizzari, & Wyss, 1971; Niedermeyer, 1972; Strobos & Kavallinis, 1968). Apparently the dynamic asymmetry of the VEP relates to the same class of phenomena. And the puzzling result obtained here shows that the abnormalities of reactivity gravitate toward the subdominant hemisphere. This preference is also revealed in an analysis of the configuration of the VEP, which evolved more frequently into wave–spike shapes or acquired an abnormally slow and simplified form on the right.

Is dynamic asymmetry really some "migrating" process that has not found its anatomic boundaries, or is it a reflection of different degrees of activity of lesions in both hemispheres? Whatever the cause of this phenomenon, it may be associated with the specific activity of the hemispheres, in some cases intensifying, in others suppressing, abnormal rhythmicity. Thus, even during normal activity of the hemispheres (or where they are equally damaged), impulses from the hypothetical subcortical lesion will be modulated depending on the level of excitability of the hemisphere, which changes, as we saw, depending on the nature of the immediate task and the time of day.

Does this mean that the specific features of hemispheric activity can be a factor determining the orientation of the lesion and the place of its final consolidation?

The information on the dynamics of VEPs may give the impression that right-sided lesions are more regular in petit mal epilepsy than in the other forms. Indeed, the material grouped in Table 4-6, which includes patients considered in the preceding section (I refer here to stationary foci disclosed on the basis of repeated EEG studies), shows that in persons suffering solely from petit mal seizures the focal epileptic process localizes most frequently on the right. When absences were combined with seizures of other types, the epileptic defect was encountered more frequently on the left. In general the number of persons having petit mal seizures showing right-sided foci is practically identical to the number showing left-sided foci.

The data in Table 4-6 are too few and statistically insignificant (binomial distribution test) to warrant far-reaching conclusions. Yet they create the impression that left-sided lesions (or involvement of the left hemisphere) are less

TABLE 4-6. Laterality of Epilepsy and Types of Seizures

Focus location	Petit mal only (number of cases)	Petit mal with history of other attacks (number of cases)
Right	5	6
Left	3	9

favorable for a prognosis of petit mal epilepsy. Even if this material is not adequate for drawing conclusions, it is sufficient to pose the question.

It will be remembered that the value of the EEG examination is problematic as regards prognosis of petit mal epilepsy. According to Gibberd (1966), whose data were based on an analysis of 139 patients, there was a strong correlation between abnormal background activity in the EEG and the occurrence of grand mal. This result coincides with our experience. Yet Charlton and Yahr (1967), who studied a larger amount of material, were skeptical: They considered the EEG an ambiguous indicator and maintained that its significance in this respect has yet to be proven.

We believe now that it is not merely the presence of pathology in the EEG, but the hemispheric orientation of the abnormality, the type of electrical activity, and the degree of recruitment of both hemispheres into the organization of epileptic activity that should be considered a prognostic criterion.

5

Factors of Hypersynchronization

WAVE–SPIKE DISCHARGES: CENTRENERGETIC OR CENTRASTHENIC?

Aristotle (cited according to Temkin, 1945) knew that epileptic seizures emerge most frequently during sleep. The probability of the appearance of paroxysmal activity when falling asleep is so significant that natural and narcotic sleep are successfully used in clinics along with other methods of discharge activation for the diagnosis of epilepsy (Fuster, 1953; Gibbs & Gibbs, 1947).

Zammarchi, Luti, and Salvatori (1967) observed petit mal seizures during active wakefulness in only 12 patients out of 32, whereas they found the seizures during sleep in 30 patients. For comparison, it should be mentioned that hyperventilation helped provoke seizures in only 22 patients. According to some observations the ratio of daytime seizures to nighttime seizures is 81:19 for grand mal seizures but 54:43 for absences (Sal y Rosas, 1952).

Most authors found that the probability of W–S discharges increases during orthodox sleep, as distinct from REM sleep, which leads to their suppression (Niedermeyer, 1965, 1966; Ross, Johnson, & Walter, 1966), although there are certain differences in the evaluation of the most vulnerable stage of slow-wave sleep. Patry, Lyagoubi, and Tassinari (1971) reported six cases observed for a number of years in whom slow-wave sleep regularly evoked an electrographical status of petit mal seizures. The discharges stopped only on waking or during the time of REM sleep. Admittedly, in one case paradoxical sleep did not stop the W–S-type complexes, but the authors especially noted that they were not certain that this was a genuine paradoxical sleep.

During slow-wave sleep, as we have seen, the SN substitutes for the AD in the VEP (Figure 4-7). The SN duration varies depending on the depth of sleep—the deeper the sleep, the greater its amplitude and duration. It is therefore thought that the appearance of petit mal seizures is facilitated in the initial stages of sleep (B–C) when the duration of the SN does not exceed 150–250 msec and when the LR emerges. Indeed, there are data to show that W–S discharges emerge in a state of light drowsiness, whereas during deep (slow) sleep only short series of spikes and waves are registered (Cadilhac & Passouant, 1964).

If the SN of the VEP in a normal sleeping person and in an epileptic patient are a reflection of deep intracortical IPSPs, as is the SN of a rabbit VEP, this reorganization of the evoked reaction may be the first stage, which under unfavorable circumstances (epilepsy, encephalopathy, and so forth) will be followed by activation of repeated W–S complexes.

Such W–S afterdischarges, resembling the EAD, were recorded only in cases where the amplitude of the SN was sufficient to be also revealed in the EEG ink records. Hence, reactivation of repeated W–S discharges is more likely in the initial stages of sleep, when the K-complex appears (Niedermeyer, 1966), which sometimes resembles a W–S discharge. Niedermeyer (1966) maintains that K-complexes serve as "physiological initiators" or even as "vehicles" of generalized or bilateral synchronous seizure discharge. The K-complex is closely associated with slow-wave sleep; epileptiform W–S discharges also appear in wakefulness. In this case what are the "physiological initiators"? If we consider abnormal rhythms in epilepsy as fragments of sleep, then is it possible that episodic W–S discharges are connected with K-complexes that should be registered in epileptics in a waking state? Perhaps the SN, which is the common component of the abnormal wave–spike VEP and of the K-complex, will in the future serve as the basis for the identification of the regular K-complex of wakefulness in epilepsy.

In any case, the appearance of paroxysmal epileptiform rhythms coincides with a feeling of tiredness, sleepiness, a certain dazedness. In a number of cases (see Table 4-3) patients and their relatives emphasized that seizures frequently emerged in daytime precisely during such periods. Patient G. V. successfully went in for sports, ran, and swam. On the advice of his physician he gave up swimming, later also running, and confined himself only to morning exercises. He noticed that this led to an increase in the frequency of seizures.

Patient B. L., who had no less than 100 seizures a day, was never subjected to them on the skating rink, where he engaged enthusiastically in figure skating. Another patient, B. A., had his first seizures at the age of 8, and by 22 they had increased to 50–70 (sometimes up to 150) per day. The patient, a student, was compelled to give up his studies because he could not master the material he heard at lectures. He felt somewhat better during practical training, but seizures stopped completely when he played chess (it was his hobby and he was a high-ranked player), especially when the game was interesting.

Patient P., a teacher at a military academy, did not take treatment for epilepsy and was not registered in any hospital, fearing that he would be dismissed from the army if the nature of his disease were known. His fears assumed neurotic proportions and he went, finally, to see a physician. It appeared that the patient was terrified of the onset of a seizure during a lecture, since this would reveal his disease. Not once did he have a seizure during a lecture, but he experienced them after his classes when in a state of relief from having completed his lecture seizure-free. The patient was visited twice by inspectors, and it is interesting to note that after their visits he no longer experienced seizures after lectures. But fits reappeared in both cases several days after he found out that the inspectors had submitted favorable reports. The patient was equally apprehensive when an EEG recording was made. After several repeated recordings his seizure accidentally registered when the technician told him that the recording session was over and asked him to wait a few moments until he would be free to remove the electrodes.

Patient M. P., on his own initiative, recorded the time of the onset of seizures for practically a year. The number of seizures was minimal during working days and sharply increased when he returned from work or was taking a nap after lunch. The number was also larger during the morning hours when he was still sluggish, sleepy, and "unable to pull himself together." Small wonder, therefore, that this patient experienced the greatest number of seizures during his vacation, when he spent more time in passive rest and sleep (Figure 5-1).

Vidart and Geier (1967) described two cases where telemetric EEG registration in hospital conditions was used to demonstrate a considerable decrease in slow waves in the EEG during the concentration of attention and mental tension. Telemetric registration was also used for the same purpose by Bureau, Guey, Dravet, and Roger (1968), who studied the EEG of 19 children between the ages of 6 and 14. They found that the most favorable conditions for the onset of a

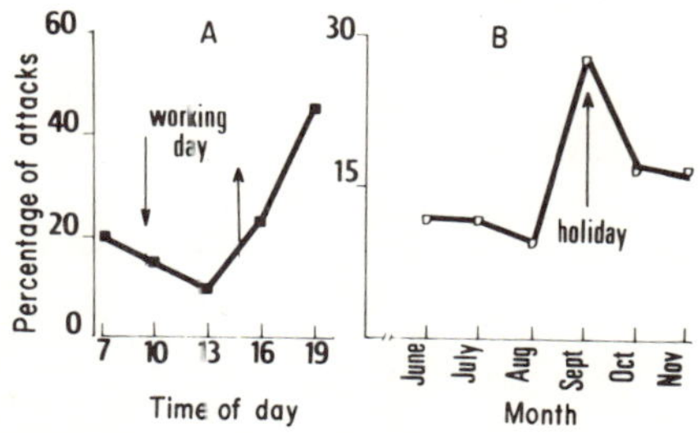

FIGURE 5-1. Incidence of petit mal fits in patient P. M. A, in daytime, and B, distribution of attacks over a 6-month period. Data collected by the patient himself.

seizure were created when the children were inactive or engaged in monotonous or boring games or work. Seizures occurred approximately four times as often as during lessons requiring mental effort, even though they could become more frequent as a result of tiredness after excessive strain.

There are also other observations that show that mental strain and active work obstruct the emergence of seizures, and if the latter do emerge, they do so predomonantly at night (Kruglova & Rubinova, 1968). Thus the view expressed by Speransky in 1932 that "the basic parts of the nervous mechanisms of sleep and an epileptic seizure are of the same nature" seems surprisingly up to date.

The probability of petit mal seizures also increases after administration of a number of drugs that synchronize the electrical activity of the cortex. Chlorpromazine in therapeutic doses not only acts as a sedative but also promotes epileptiform activity and W–S-type discharges, both in epileptics and in virtually healthy persons (Ekiert & Bigo, 1959). Some authors maintain that as regards its ability to activate epileptic discharges in the EEG, it competes with such potent convulsants as Metrazol.

This aspect of the action of chlorpromazine may be connected with its suppressive action on the desynchronizing abilities of the reticular formation. Schefer and Fuks (1969) noted that in treating hypothalamic epilepsy it is not advisable to use drugs that block the activating reticular formation. Evidently, sedative drugs should be used with greater caution in the treatment of epilepsy, especially of petit mal forms.

Further, it was experimentally established here that spontaneous W–S-type discharges emerge after destruction of the subthalamus and the mesencephalic reticular formation. This also lowers the threshold of the appearance of convulsive activity in response to Metrazol injections.

The destruction of various brain-stem areas leads to considerable intensification of activity in a previously created but dormant epileptic focus. This, too, leads to myoclonic and generalized seizures, and the development of 3-per-second W–S discharges in the EEG (Stevens *et al.*, 1964). Milhorat *et al.* (1966) recommend lesions in the rostral part of the reticular formation to obtain a stable model of a myoclonic epileptic seizure.

It is well known that the reticular formation exerts a suppressive action on convulsive discharges of the W–S type (Lennox, 1960; Guerrero-Figueroa *et al.*, 1963a, b). Hence, the destruction of the oral pole of the brain stem leads to a considerable lowering of the threshold of inhibitory epileptiform rhythms. Tumors of deep cerebral structures and the cerebellum may lead to W–S paroxysms (Madsen & Bray, 1966). This is true with one proviso. Although stimulation of the reticular formation, as also the injection of sympathomimetics, suppresses the SN and derivative forms of synchronized and hypersynchronized oscillations in rabbits, the SN is not blocked against the background of desynchronization evoked by galanthamine (Nivalin), an inhibitor of cholinesterase. This drug also leads to a sharp increase of the LR and provokes the EAD; this reminds one of the action of Metrazol, which also desynchronizes the EEG. It may be that the arousal of cholinenergic origin not only fails to block W–S-type complexes, but even facilitates their development by acting on the "rebound" mechanisms on which the LR is based.

In describing the effect of damage of brain-stem structures on the emergence of experimental W–S discharges, I noted that the desynchronization of the EEG, which formerly suppressed the EAD, becomes ineffective after surgery. This phenomenon was particularly clearly expressed following damage to the dorsal part of the brain stem and led to the belief that some other type of arousal reaction was unmasked, one possessing other properties. Indeed, the experimental animals did not manifest any symptoms of behavioral activation during the onset of desynchronization, which resembles the classical effect of the dissociation of the EEG pattern and behavior following injection of M-cholinergic physostigmine (Bradley, 1958).

Perhaps the morphological basis of these effects may be an ascending cholinergic reticular system (Shute & Lewis, 1967). It was shown previously that tetanization of the nonspecific structures blocks W–S discharges and SN–LR complexes. Considering the genesis of the SN, we may speak of the ability of reticular impulses to block and desynchronize the process of postsynaptic inhibition. Apparently, suppression of IPSPs is connected with the lowering of the effectiveness of inhibitory synaptic action.

Purpura *et al.* (1966) explained the blockade of the IPSP of thalamic neurons during tetanization of the brain-stem reticular formation by assuming that impulses from the reticular structures activate specialized elements that exert a depressing action on inhibitory interneurons ("inhibition of inhibition") and/or blockade presynaptically inhibitory cells or some excitatory elements that have an activating effect on them.

Skrebitsky (1967) compared the VEP to the intracellularly recorded activity of visual neurons on the background of auditory stimulation. He observed a decrease in the amplitudes and duration of IPSPs against the background of sound, coinciding with the suppression of the SN and the LR. He, too, believes that this effect is associated with the blockade of the activity of inhibitory interneurons or may be due to presynaptic inhibition.

It has already been mentioned that low-frequency stimulation of the caudate nucleus evokes the SN, and a typical arrest reaction develops. During extracellular recording of the activity of cortical cells it was noticed that they stop firing during the SN for 150–250 msec (Buchwald *et al.,* 1967). Hull *et al.* (1967) showed that the period of the suppression of spike activity also corresponds with an IPSP. A combination of stimulation of the caudate nucleus with any afferent stimulus (Hull *et al.* used LGB stimulation) led to suppression of the arrest reaction, decreased the period of IPSP in the cortical cells, and led to the disappearance of rebound discharges. For example, disinhibition was observed during stimulation of the geniculate body when stimulation occurred 50–100 msec after the electric shock delivered to the caudate nucleus. It was interesting that the phenomenon was universal; it was also recorded when stimulating nonspecific thalamic nuclei (Buchwald *et al.,* 1967).

It has been mentioned previously that the removal of reticulothalamic influences increases the duration of the secondary SN, EAD, and SEAD. Similar phenomena were described by other writers following neuronal isolation of cortical islets (Schlag, 1966) and removal or suppression of the activity of diencephalic structures (Naquet *et al.,* 1964).

Apparently, an extension of the SN may result from asynchronous IPSPs of normal duration and/or the intensification of postsynaptic inhibition. Here, the increase of the duration of the SN is accompanied by a substantial facilitation of the LR amplitude and the emergence of the EAD and the SEAD. This is apparently impossible with asynchronous IPSPs—which is an argument for the development of a hypersynchronous process. This assumption was also supported by extracellular and quasi-intracellular records in cortical cells of ir-radiated animals showing long-lasting SN. Hence, the IPSP amplitudes in the cortex increase substantially.

Since presynaptic inhibitory input from the reticular formation may decrease the duration and the amplitude of cortical and subcortical IPSPs, it is tempting to assume that an increase of postsynaptic hyperpolarization occurs because of the removal of presynaptic reticular influences, which control the activity of the cortical elements either directly or through some intermediate structures. It is not impossible that the reticular formation influences the cortex through the thalamic relay nuclei. However, despite the information outlined here, it seems rather improbable if we consider the phenomenon of reticular blockade of the postsynaptic components of cortical responses to stimulation of the visual radiation. The latter showed virtually no changes following destruction of the lateral geniculate body (Courtois & Cordeau, 1969). Unfortunately, there is no precise information on the circuit of elements in which this process is at work.

But in any case the nature of inhibitory hypersynchronization and correspondingly of petit mal potentials is indeed *centrasthenic* rather than *centrenergetic.* Since the reticular formation is able to inhibit the excessive expression of postsynaptic inhibition, we should add, taking into account the data we have about the effect of inhibitory hypersynchronies on behavior, that we are dealing with a unique sensory hunger, a sensory underemployment of the cortex, which is a factor promoting the organization of W–S autorhythmicity. In this situation any subcortical structure or structures released for similar reasons from reticular control are able to become pacemakers of hypersynchronous cortical activity, if their afferents reach the cortex.

PLEASURE RHYTHM AS A PRECURSOR OF WAVE–SPIKE ACTIVITY

With the exception of the special role of presynaptic control of cortical activity, the explanations of the formation of hypersynchronous regular rhythms discussed previously were based on traditional ideas about the unbalancing of cortical–subcortical relations extended to mechanisms for the organization of hypersynchronous activity. This assumption is based on premises about the unique nature of the energetic, desynchronizing abilities of the reticular system, and on its ability to control convulsive rhythms, which has been sufficiently well argued (Okujava, 1969). The number of structures known to be capable of desynchronizing electrical activity has grown considerably since it was noticed that the effect of activation is as dependent on the frequency of stimulation as it is on the specificity of the centers stimulated.

Closer scrutiny shows that discussing a lowering of tonus by activating the reticular system was only justified in general. Most of the areas whose destruction evokes synchronization of electrical activity and W–S discharges, such as the central gray matter, habenular nuclei, dorsal hypothalamus, and subthalamus, are part of the limbic system or are very closely linked with it. Additional consideration of the limbic system greatly complicates the centrasthenic hypothesis of the genesis of hypersynchronous activity, and it becomes necessary to consider the mechanisms of sleep, wakefulness, and the organization of convulsive rhythms in relation to the mechanisms of the graduation and organization of emotional reactions.

When electroencephalographic changes are taken as the criteria, it is found that the limbic system reproduces the effects of the reticular formation, for the latter can be considered its addressee. For the reticular formation "the aim is nothing, while movement is everything," whereas the limbic centers "know" what they want to achieve and, moreover, are programmed to attain their aim. Thus, synchronization of the EEG may be achieved equally by damage to the executive mechanisms of activation, which are then unable to activate the cortex and other centers, and by damage to the command apparatus of the drive system, causing the brain to sink into sleep due to the absence of motivation.

It may not be a coincidence that the areas evoking synchronization and hypersynchronization of the EEG are located in the limbic midbrain area: the region of central gray, the periventricular system, the dorsolateral perifornical area, and the subthalamus. These are structures that relate to the "punishment system" or, in other words, structures whose stimulation evokes drive. In this sense the areas marked in black in Figures 1-17 and 1-21 coincide with those of negative reinforcement in maps given by Bruner (1967) and Black and Vanderwolf (1969). Animals seek to decrease the activity of this system, despite the seeming paradox that the highest rates of self-stimulation are registered in some of these punishment zones.

The stimulation of the central gray matter in the midbrain evokes all the symptoms of a defensive reaction, ranging from fear to aggression (Halpern, 1968), and naturally animals quickly learn instrumental behaviors to escape from electric stimulation of this area of the brain (Cooper & Taylor, 1967). The whole set of vegetative reactions accompanying stimulation testifies to the activation of the ergotrophic system.

Depending on the size of the injury, destruction of the periaqueductal gray matter in rabbits, cats, and rats produces a lowering of locomotor activity, drowsiness, disturbance of the avoidance reaction, deterioration of orienting, decreased reactivity to external stimuli including pain and so on (Halpern, 1968); Skultety, 1958). These are all phenomena resembling those we described following similar destructions of the central aqueductal gray matter in rabbits and rats. According to Adey (1958) a decrease in reaction to painful stimuli in baboons and phalangers following removal of the entorhinal cortex is related to a disturbance of the afferents between the hypothalamus and the central gray matter. The disappearance of affective reaction in cats in response to stimulation of the paraventricular nucleus of the hypothalamus following destruction of the central gray matter (Skultety, 1958) may also be connected with a deterioration of the regulation of reactions to pain stimuli. This would be effected through the dorsal longitudinal bundle of Schutz, a system of fibers beginning at the ventral part of the periaqueductal gray matter, partially ending in the intralaminar thalamic nuclei, but mainly terminating in the caudal section of the periventricular area.

Stimulation of the habenular nucleus, as well as the central gray matter, is perceived by the animal as a "punishment." A single electric shock in that area associated with a lever press will disrupt a well-established instrumental feeding reaction in a cat, and it cannot be restored even after 3 days of hunger (Doti, 1958). In the same way destruction of the habenular nuclei destroys regulation of behavior in a stressful situation, lowers locomotor activity, and diminishes the avoidance reaction (Nielson & McIver, 1966). For the time being it is difficult to explain these effects, but it should be borne in mind that among the lateral afferents in the limbic system–midbrain circuit the system of fibers emerging from the habenula (habenulopeduncular tract) holds an important place. In addition to projections to the interpeduncular nucleus they spread laterally and embrace an extensive area of the brain stem (Nauta, 1960). When the habenula is destroyed, degenerating fibers are found in the central gray matter of the midbrain, the superior colliculi, and the thalamic intralaminar nuclei (Katsuhito & Powell, 1968).

Stimulation of the zona incerta also leads to a sort of "one-trial learning"; after a single lever press an animal will never again repeat self-stimulation (Olds,

1960). It is not possible that the participation of this formation in the regulation of affective reactions is not so much connected with its nonspecific tonigenic influence on the cortex and its ability to modulate the activity of the mesencephalic reticular formation, as with its specific role as one of the "hunger centers" in the realization of feeding behavior (Miller, 1961). When stimulating this area in a rabbit we observed an abrupt behavioral and electrographic arousal reaction with chaotic locomotor—exploratory behavior and thumping. These were sometimes evoked by lower intensities of current than used in stimulation of the central gray matter.

It therefore seems natural that destruction of the subthalamus, as well as the central gray matter, leads to apathy, areactivity, disturbance of the avoidance reaction, and, because of the predominance of the tonus of synchronizing "trophotrophic" zones, to a slowing down of the electrical activity of the brain, the external variant of which may possibly be wave—spike-type hypersynchrony. A typical feature of the experiments by Adey (1958), mentioned previously, was that monkeys with removed entorhinal areas became tender and accessible. They did not display their usual aggression in contacts with the experimenter. Along with this, a stimulus with a latent period on the order of 300 msec led to the emergence of afteractivity in the auditory cortex.

Synchronized activity does not emerge only during the coarse suppression of ergotrophic mechanisms. It is a concomitant of the selective satisfaction of the organism's main requirements. Porter, Cavanaugh, Critchlow, and Sawyer (1957) observed that during mechanical vaginal stimulation of estrous cats paroxysmal bursts of synchronized activity occurred in the lateral hypothalamus at a frequency near the sigma and theta band. According to Sawyer's group (Sawyer, 1960; Sawyer & Kawakami, 1959) vaginal stimulation in rabbits and rats evokes high-voltage, low-frequency activity in the cortex resembling the rhythmicity of slow-wave sleep and sometimes activity similar to W—S. An identical rhythmicity is described by Sutin and Michael (1970) as an aftereffect of vaginal stimulation.

Porter and Bors (1962) observed synchronization of the EEG in cats following a sudden reduction of pressure in the bladder after it had been overfilled. This synchronization attained so high a voltage that it would not be an exaggeration to speak of its evolution into seizure rhythmicity.

Sudakov (1965) showed that feeding a hungry animal or injecting glucose replaces desynchronized ("hungry") activity in the frontal areas of the cortex and lateral hypothalamic nuclei with slow activity. This effect, repeatedly substantiated by other authors at a later data, was named by Morgane (1969) *satiated sleep.*

In cats trained to press a lever for milk following several reinforcements bursts of high-amplitude 4—8-per-second waves developed in the primary and secondary visual areas during the lever presses and while the cats were drinking the milk (Clemente, Sterman, & Wyrwicka, 1964; Hackett *et al.,* 1971). This *postrein-*

forcement synchronization, as it was called by the authors, stabilized fully at the end of the experiment. In some cases the form of the oscillations and their frequency greatly resembled exalted W–S afterdischarges in the visual cortex of rabbits. Naturally, such hypersynchronous activity is an excellent background for the development of seizures.

Before I discuss the pathophysiological implications of this model let me stress that the term *postreinforcement synchronization* (Clemente *et al.,* 1964) was introduced to designate only the consequences of some specific behavioral situation. It should therefore apparently be further specified, since identical waves also develop in a satiated, drowsy animal in a familiar safe situation, with a low probability of awakening stimuli. Behavioral studies by my group (previously described) and the studies of Livanov (1962) and Roitbak (1960) show that a burst of synchronizing activity develops following termination of a defensive reinforcement. This is essentially equivalent to a reward (withdrawal from the painful situation), but with respect to this reflex it may be called *nonreinforcement synchronization.* As many terms may be suggested for this phenomenon as there are situations evoking it, but it is typical of them all that the animal finds itself in a comfortable or safe situation, at rest, satiated with respect to sex and food. It may therefore be advisable to call regular activity of this type *pleasure rhythms* (Myslobodsky, 1970a).

Piontkovsky (1964) described antenatally irradiated pups in whom seizures, which were often lethal, developed exclusively during feedings. Scollo-Lavizzari and Hess (1967) report the onset of epileptic seizures in a boy during eating, but it is difficult to assume that such cases are developed against the background of postreinforcement synchronization. Nevertheless, these facts have a wider significance—they refer us to the old question about the role of emotions in the pathogenesis of an epileptic seizure. Admittedly, the fact that emotional disturbances are a frequent concomitant of epilepsy has been known for so long that interest in this fact has somewhat flagged. In clinics, emotional states are constantly revealed that constitute part of the aura of the onset of the seizure. During epileptic rhythms a state of violent sexual excitement may develop (Ohtani, Hirano, & Kita, 1962), bordering on orgasm (Patarnello, 1963). In other cases there may be a nondifferentiated feeling of joy, pacification, and harmony, an unusual feeling of fullness, satisfaction, serenity, and all-comprehension, similar to the moments preceding the fits experienced by Count Myshkin in Dostoevski's *The Idiot.*

Some .1% of people suffering from epilepsy (Andermann, Berman, Cooke, Dickson, Gastaut, Kennedy, Margerison, Pond, Tizard, & Walsh, 1962) discovered for themselves that flickering is able to evoke seizures and may be accompanied by a feeling of pleasure. It is difficult to obtain precise descriptions of what they experience since they are generally children with serious intellectual defects. They deliberately evoke fits by looking at a bright light source, such as the sun or a lamp, and waving their hands before their eyes, shaking their head, or blinking. These fits generally take the form of petit mal seizures, although there are also reports of grand mal convulsive fits evolving from absence. Many authors believe that these self-stimulated seizures evoke a pleasure similar to that experienced by animals during brain self-stimulation with an electric current. In any case, some children refuse to wear sunglasses, which prevent seizures. It would seem that self-provoked photogenic seizures are a payment made by the brain for the pleasure evoked by the synchronizing action of flickering light. Other ways of provoking voluntary and nonvoluntary epileptic discharges have been described, such as deep and frequent breathing, which may occur during smoking, masturbation, or sexual orgasm (Fabisch & Darbyshire, 1965; Hoenig & Hamilton, 1960; Mosovich & Tallaferro, 1954; Van Reeth, 1959).

Generally, positive emotions are far more frequent concomitants of fits than could be suspected from their external expression—tears, anger, and aggression. In many patients even such negative affects can produce a pleasant feeling. The activation of the reward zones may be accompanied, as we saw, by synchronization of electrical activity. Thus, if hypersynchronous rhythms of the W–S type are the cause of a positive emotional "accompaniment" of epileptic seizures, it is not impossible that positive emotions in epileptics may evoke seizures. Yet, reports of the association of seizures with negative emotion and shock are far more frequent (Gowers, 1885; Sepp *et al.,* 1947). It is because of its drama that this correlation was recognized as regular and natural. Grand mal seizures generally develop in these cases and the behavioral manifestations are clear and impressive. Such a correlation may be understood as the outcome of the activation of zones of negative reinforcement, creating a desynchronized background against which the paroxysms of a hyperdepolarizing genesis should emerge or be facilitated in predisposed persons. Something similar takes place in animals irradiated on the twenty-third day of embryogenesis, when the lowering of the threshold of the electroconvulsive afterdischarge correlates with desynchronization of the EEG background and an increase in behavioral activity. It was shown experimentally that against the background of Metrazol or picrotoxin poisoning, tetanization of the posterior hypothalamus or reticular formation or administration of painful stimulation intensifies convulsive discharges to the extent that they resemble the rhythmicity typical of grand mal convulsive seizures in humans (Gellhorn & Loofborrow, 1963). Hence, it seems that one should seek examples of the provocation of hypersynchronous activity by positive emotions in the group of petit mal seizures.

Some time ago, a connection was suspected between the phenomenon of self-stimulation and epileptiform episodes as a sign of general elevation of brain excitability. However, a check showed that self-stimulation was accompanied by convulsive afterdischarges only when it was enduring, and the current intensity was sufficient to induce repeated brain stimulation (Bogacz, St. Laurent, & Olds, 1965). The impression was created that the seizure was a consequence of excessive and enduring stimulation, and not of an anatomic coincidence of low-threshold zones with areas of positive reinforcement, as Olds believed (1960). This ended the discussion about the epileptic discharge as a substratum of the effect of self-stimulation, and later it was shown that repeated self-stimulation even leads to a resistence to fits (Herberg, Tress, & Blundell, 1969).

Yet, this cannot be considered a valid conclusion, primarily because it is based on a study in which electrical activity during self-stimulation episodes and 1–2 sec following their termination was distorted by artifacts of the stimulating current. Hence, the studies of Bogacz *et al.* (1965) indicate there is no connection between self-stimulation and grand mal seizures, but this does not relate to phenomena of the absence type. In this respect the argument against Olds' assumption seems quite justified since he presupposed that epileptic reactions emerged against a background of high level of neuronal excitation. Even the use of a criterion such as the threshold of the convulsive afterdischarge evoked by direct stimulation indicates reference is being made to a rhythmicity typical of grand mal seizures.

Indeed, the data discussed earlier contain an interesting suggestion that the activity of the positive zones may even *suppress* seizures of the hyperdepolarization type, such as grand mal, because of the ability of the reward system to synchronize the EEG. That is why during repetitive self-stimulation sessions a resistance to grand mal fits may build up, even if they were previously readily evoked by excessive stimulation of the same electrode. This may have been the case in the experiments carried out by Herberg *et al.* (1969).

The view of self-stimulation as a phenomenon increasing brain excitability gained ground, especially when it was found that an animal may also work to obtain a puff of air, smells, sound stimulations, changes in the illumination of the chamber, and even moderate electrical stimulation of the skin (Berlyne, 1969), but there are many explanations for these facts. On the whole, it seems natural to interpret them as an indication that the organism can strive for an increase of its energetic potential, for "drive induction" (Sheffield, 1966).

In 1960 Olds conventionally divided the elements of the brain into three classes:

1. Cells, toward the excitation of which the body strives, and which, to judge from the extensive spread of reward zones, account for 35% of the total.
2. Cells, the excitation of which it avoids. These comprise 5% of the total.
3. Cells, toward the excitation of which the organism does not strive or avoid, i.e., neutral elements or zones. These predominate and account for 60%.

The predominance of pleasure zones over punishment zones suggested that the brain cannot be thought of as tending mainly to produce behaviors which decrease its own excitation, for the onset of stimulation in large regions of the brain produces behavior which increases excitation (Olds, 1960).

This view, however, is by no means self-evident. Emergence of a drive is easily demonstrated in the presence of the goal–object during stimulation of the same brain zones that animal seeks to self-stimulate (Valenstein, 1969). Therefore, it could be that self-stimulation is directed at lowering the drive, to reduce the brain energetic potential. This is especially likely since the rate of self-stimulation for the corresponding brain areas is inversely proportional to the degree of the animal's satiation with food (Hoebel, 1962) and sex (Caggiula, 1970). These facts could, however, be accepted as indicators of a stable anatomic organization of the drive system, if one were sure that the rate of self-stimulation of other brain zones does not change under the effect of hunger or hormonal intervention (Valenstein, 1969). At the same time Hodos and Valenstein (1960) demonstrated that hunger increases the rate of self-stimulation of the septum, the tetanization of which does not produce feeding behavior. By the way, thirst and hunger have the same influence on the rate of lever pressing, as do stimuli considered indifferent (Berlyne, 1969). It would seem that an arousal reaction of any origin leads to identical consequences (Lilly, 1960).

In experiments made with Kuznetsova (Myslobodsky & Kuznetsova, 1971) a study was made of self-stimulation by light. Nine rats of the Wistar line were placed in a box of organic glass, 20 X 30 X 25 cm, which contained a pedal on one wall. Pedal presses activated a brief (50 msec) light flash (.3 joule). The strobe was placed above the box and, generally, paired stimuli with an interval of 150 msec were used.

In experimental sessions where the pedal did not produce light flashes the rats stopped responding altogether and showed no preference for any part of the chamber. When the light stimulator was switched on, it became clear by the second or third session that the animal deliberately and purposely pressed the lever and preferred to sit on the pedal or near it between presses. Over 200 experiments made with these animals established that the frequency of pressing varied from 20 to 150 per hour, never, however, exceeding 200 per hour; after 30–50 min the rat stopped pressing the pedal and fell asleep.

Stimulation by pain or the injection of Phenamine (d-amphetamine) intensified the rate of self-stimulation. Doses of 2–5 mg/kg amphetamine were introduced intraperitoneally. Injections of isotonic sodium chloride solution served as control. A total of 30 experiments in nine rats were made with the drug.

Some minutes following injection the animals became more mobile and fussy, and the number of pedal presses decreased somewhat. However, 5–20 min later self-stimulations sharply increased in six out of nine rats, and sometimes exceeded the initial level by several dozen (Figure 5-2). When the pedal was disconnected from the light, pressing quickly stopped, although the animals periodically effected "test" presses.

It is not excluded that light self-stimulation is connected with the activity of the classical centers of positive reinforcement, for it is known that the medial forebrain bundle in the rat contains a central visual projection, the inferior accessory optic tract.

Later, Konnikov (1974), a student of mine, tested the possibility of self-stimulation of the lateral geniculate body. He discovered statistically significant self-stimulation in 13 rats out of 17 studied. In all rats it took the form of relatively short (1–3 min) approaches to the pedal, accompanied by vigorous pressing, the frequency of which sometimes reached 1600 per hour. During the experiment most of the animals made 8–12 such runs; hence, the summary rate of pressing during the entire experiment did not exceed 300 per hour, which is within the limits of the rate for light self-stimulation. This type of self-stimulation did not change fundamentally when the intensity of the stimulating current was doubled, although noticeable motor effects of electric stimulation appeared. In fact, it was found that when higher currents were used, the cyclic nature of self-stimulation was emphasized, and its rate could increase. Generally when the intensity of the stimuli was higher, the animal, following several ferocious presses, froze near the pedal or jumped away from it and then began a new series of presses with the same ferocity. In the intervals between presses the animal fell into a doze on the pedal or near it. When the current was switched off, the rats quickly stopped pressing. Thus a specific sensory center seemed to have properties considered unique to some hypothalamic limbic centers.

The hypothalamus is considered a sort of conglomerate of anatomically separate systems controlling various drives, which, it seemed, was corroborated by the effect of stimulation. However, in the strictly controlled studies made in Valenstein's laboratory, no clear evidence was found for rigid connections of particular drives with discrete sections of the hypothalamus. Valenstein writes:

> the diversity of sites capable of eliciting carrying behavior suggests that no specific hypothalamic area mediates this behavior and the possibility exists that the behavior is organised elsewhere in the nervous system. To the extent that it may be appropriate to generalize to other stimulus-bound behavior, it would appear more profitable to view the behavior elicited by hypothalamic stimulation as prepotent responses initiated by interaction of "general states" and environmental conditions prior to the postulation of motivational states related to biological needs. *The term "general states" is not meant to imply that it will not be possible to differentiate the effects of stimulation at different hypothalamic regions, but rather that the application of specific terms such as hunger, thirst and sex may not be justified* [Valenstein, 1969, p. 300].

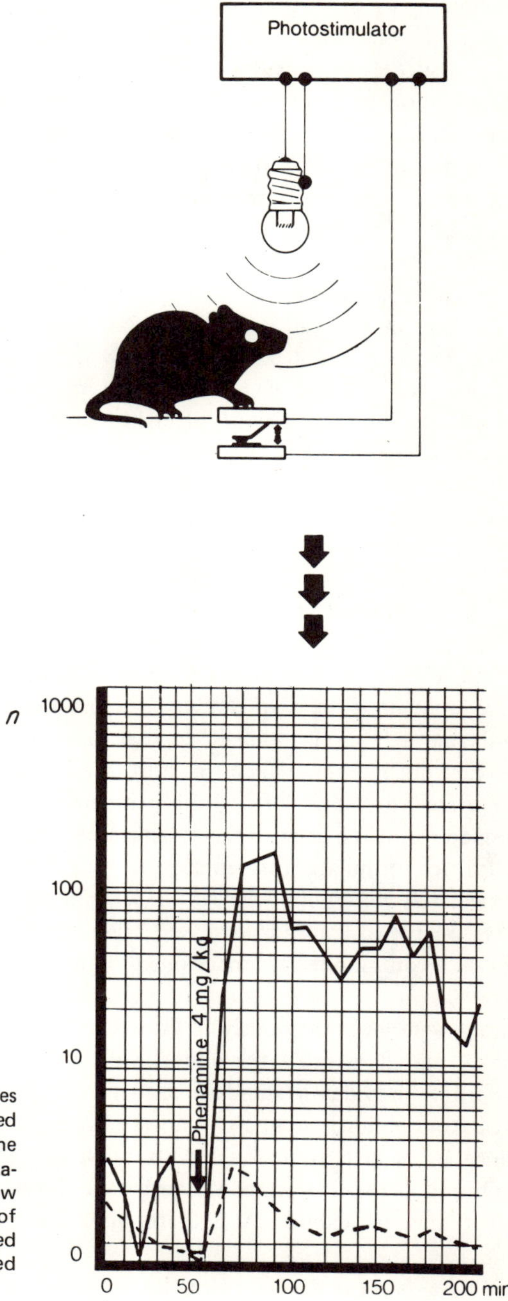

FIGURE 5-2. Number of bar-presses (*n*) for light stimuli in nontreated white rats (broken line) and after the injection of 4 mg/kg of d-amphetamine (Phenamine) (solid line). Arrow on the graph marks the time of Phenamine injection in the treated rat and saline injection in nontreated rat.

In summing up the experiments cited here, Valenstein wrote that "specific predictions of evoked behavior based on anatomical locus would have a low probability of success [Valenstein, 1969, p. 313]."

Stimulation of structures of the human brain including the hypothalamus may evoke emotional shifts, but it does so by producing agitation, fear, apprehension, or, on the other hand, increased socializing, euphoria, and relaxation, but no hint of any specific motivational state (Delgado, 1969; Heath, 1954; Sem-Jacobsen & Torkildsen, 1960). There are reasons to believe that high-frequency electrical stimulation of the centers evokes conditions that may be described as an inexplicable undifferentiated appetite, desire, or fear. Self-stimulation is then in the same measure an act of reduction of a modally nonspecific drive. Recently Stutz, Butcher, and Rossi (1969) proved that an animal does not distinguish between the effects of reinforcement of two anatomically distinct positive reward zones if they do not differ in the rates of self-stimulation they sustain. Stutz *et al.* wrote: "Our findings disclose the possibility that many of the diverse structures which support self-stimulation are part of a generalized or undifferentiated reward system [1969, p. 1082]."[1] Thus, one should agree with Valenstein (1969) that the specific nature of drives is acquired at the stage of the emergence of a definite functional organization similar to a conditioned reflex.

Yet, the motivational equipotentiality of the hypothalamic centers may turn out to be illusory. It is not excluded that centers of specific drives may exist, but in the absence of conditions for the satisfaction of a particular requirement, there may be a shift of activity toward the satisfaction of any other drive attainable at a given moment. In that case we would have to admit that drives are interchangeable, which in turn predicates the existence of some single interbrain process, a sort of universal currency, which is perceived as a reward irrespective of the need of the organism being satisfied at the given moment. It is useful to formulate this conjecture in neurophysiological terms. We should immediately determine whether, in keeping with the logic of drive induction, it is reasonable to consider increased brain excitability in the sense formulated by Olds as a common reward mechanism. In my view there are grounds for a negative answer.

Data were given previously to show that in both the cortex and the subcortical nuclei, including those the animal will self-stimulate, the system of recurrent inhibition provides a standard sequence of reactions to an electric stimulus: EPSPs and action potentials, followed by the development of long-lasting IPSPs. Hence, it is just as reasonable to think of self-stimulation as a striving for inhibition as for excitation. Moreover, the threshold of inhibition is considerably higher than for excitation. Self-stimulation sets in at a current of considerable

---

[1] It is interesting to note that many hedonists have held that pleasures are alike, differing only in intensity and duration.

intensity, and it is known that in response to the electric stimulus long IPSPs develop in addition to EPSPs and action potentials. The duration of the IPSP is considerably longer than that of the EPSP, and perhaps the former determines phenomena such as an animal's freezing during self-stimulation, which resembles the evoked "arrest reaction" of Hunter and Jasper (1949). Thus, striving for repeated stimulation of the brain (and hence, the reward mechanism) can be expressed as striving for the development of synchronous IPSPs in the given center or subordinated structures.

Konnikov (1974) found that when the lateral geniculate was stimulated with a series of four rectangular pulses (frequency 60–100 Hz, pulse duration .5 msec), the primary reactions were registered at intensities of about 1–2 V. The SN was irregular and its duration did not exceed 100–200 μV. During that period pedal pressing was only accidental. When an increase in the stimulus to 4–5 V produced an SN with an amplitude of 200 ± 22 μV, and a duration of 118.9 ± 7.18 msec, the rat began to press the pedal regularly. Repeated research disclosed that the threshold of lateral geniculate self-stimulation can with satisfactory reliability be determined by the appearance of a stable SN. A further rise in the intensity of the stimuli to 6–7 V increased the duration of the SN to 175–190 msec (175.3 ± 21.5) and the amplitude to 300–450 μV. This frequently led to the appearance of a high-amplitude LR followed by a new SN. With the appearance of this configuration the rats approached the pedal less frequently, and self-stimulation acquired the nature of episodic ferocious "accords," ending in the characteristic cataplexy and shaking of the head. Thus active behavior per se is not necessarily an indicator of drive-induction tendency; rather, it may represent a drive for *activation of* brain sites producing long-lasting *inhibitory waves* and rebound discharges. Paradoxically enough, then, drive induction may be an instrument of drive reduction.

The IPSP may be a unique microtarget of the reward effect; excitation of nervous tissue, including the reticular formation, may actually tend to service the mechanism of drive search and mastery of the macrotarget, be it food, the female, or the pedal controlling distribution of electric current. Actually we refer not to "pure" IPSPs, but to a definite class of rhythmical activity. Provided the background excitatory synaptic activity evoked by the drive state is sufficiently high, though not high enough to eliminate IPSPs, the inhibitory synaptic action triggered by the excitation of a reward stimulus (electrical or natural) may synchronize the EEG into a pattern resembling postreinforcement synchronization—according to the theory of Eccles (1965), and Andersen and Andersson (1968).[2]

---

[2] Recently Ito (1972) found neurons of the medial forebrain bundle which were inhibited during self-stimulation of the lateral hypothalamus.

Because of the genetic unity of the considered rhythms (sensory afterdischarges) with the EAD and the SEAD, we can maintain that if self-stimulation is really accompanied by epileptiform discharges, these discharges must be related to the potentials of petit mal or, at least, to normal SN—LR complexes. Indeed, Newman and Feldman (1964) noted that spikes and slow waves are a rather constant concomitant of self-stimulation if the EEG is registered 1–2 sec following self-stimulation. This seems to correspond with the assumption about the connection of inhibitory hypersynchronies with reward mechanisms. The lowering of the self-stimulation rate following injection of Metrazol does not contradict this assumption, because Metrazol leads to the organization of W—S-type potentials or lowers the threshold for their appearance. And if paroxysmal rhythms of that type can be associated with pleasure, the presence of W—S discharges in the background EEG must decrease the striving for repeated stimulation. In other words, W—S discharges may be seen as an accentuated pleasure rhythm, an exaggerated state of drive reduction.

In view of the ideas of inhibitory synchronization as the basis of the reward system, it seems doubtful that there exists a single center of self-stimulation. It is reasonable that no such center has been found, since the structural and physical bases of reward are assumed to be local autosynchronization circuits of recurrent inhibition, i.e., a mechanism highly decentralized. This conclusion has a number of consequences, examined earlier (Myslobodsky, 1970a,b). At this time it is important to emphasize one of them. If the rhythms that are potential precursors of W—S-type complexes are able to form in any nervous center, the nature of the W—S discharge itself must be considered polycentric, as Walker and Marshall maintained (1961, 1964). One of these centers may be the centrencephalic system or virtually any section of the limbic—reticular complex. The only questions are when, under what circumstances, and how frequently such conditions are created.

For example, the synchronization centers of the hypnogenic system (anterior thalamic nuclei, preoptic area, basal ganglia, orbital cortex, and other structures) can be pacemakers if, in the presence of other factors promoting the epileptization of rhythmicity, they slip from the control of the reticular activating system.

Limbic-forebrain circuits in their turn control the reticular activating system, for they are the center where decisions are made concerning the degree of activation necessary for orienting to an external signal. They are responsible for selective modulation of different signals, activation of the motor system during the search for food, water, or a female, or during escape from a potential enemy, where the reticular activating system is mostly an executive apparatus. Hence synchronization of the EEG must also set in during a disturbance of communications between motivation centers, particularly in centers of negative reinforcement and in executive brain-stem reticular mechanisms. This creates a state of selective deafferentation or information hunger in the reticular formation, since it has no information about the organism's requirements. Because of the reticular formation's lower level of activity the subordinated centers, too, are in a state of sensory underemployment.

A consistent defense of the view that pleasure synchrony, like postreinforcement synchronization, is the precursor of human petit mal discharges is difficult because pleasure rhythms are practically absent in a normal adult person. The observations made by Mosovich and Tallaferro (1954), cited previously, are unfortunately not documented. Only the *hedonic hypersynchrony,* which emerges in the occipital derivations in a child during positive emotions (Maulsby, 1971), is related to the sensory theta-rhythm that may be the precursor of W–S discharges. It is not impossible that in the period of life when alpha rhythm is still absent or unstable, such rhythms are not rare. In adults the activity of the cortex, constrained by rhythms in the alpha range, shifts only little in the direction of synchronization during pleasure. It seems, for example, that in some cases the development of a blissful, pleasant state (Lilly & Shurley, 1961) during sensory isolation may be paralleled by a slowdown of the EEG (Zubek & Welch, 1963).

Another reason for the rarity with which the pleasure rhythm is recorded in humans may be rather technical: Authors seldom care to study the activity of both hemispheres. According to Goldstein's data cited by Fisher (1975), at the peak of sexual ecstasy (i.e., orgasm) a slow high-amplitude activity develops in the right hemisphere. The left hemisphere at this time displays a persistent preorgasmic alpha-activity.[3]

WAVE–SPIKE DISCHARGES AND
THE LAW OF DENERVATION

Sensory isolation may lead to the synchronization of electrical activity and, in the event of long-lasting action, promote the development of epileptiform disorders in the EEG.

The synchronization and hypersynchronization of the EEG may be a consequence of visual deafferentation (Novikova, 1965; Zislina & Novikova, 1971).

The suppression of proprioceptive impulses following the injection of myorelaxants also leads to a slowdown of the EEG, typical of the sleep evolution of rhythmicity (Gellhorn & Loofborrow, 1963). In unrestrained, isolated animals, sensory hunger and sensory underemployment lead to serious disturbances of the behavior and of the regulation of electrocortical activity (Melzack, 1965). It

---

[3] It was mentioned that the right hemisphere has a negative emotional charge. In a case of right-side hypersynchronization caused by subdominant pathology, barbiturization, or the development of pleasure rhythms the release of the optimistic left hemisphere may lead to an unusually high pleasure sensation. One may see such episodes in patients with temporal lobe epilepsy.

is acceptable to interpret such facts in keeping with the hypothesis of the development of supersensitivity in denervated structures (Cannon & Rosenblueth, 1949). Although it is not always beneficial to apply (or "overuse") this law, its use has become traditional for the explanation of epileptiform disorders (see Stavraky, 1961; Sharpless, 1964). In kittens kept in darkness from birth, it was extremely simple to evoke rhythmical cellular and EEG responses resembling exalted sensory afterdischarges (Satterberg & Ganz, 1967). Such afterdischarges could increase and even evolve into the rhythmicity typical of a grand mal seizure. Rosenblum (1963) found a lowering of the electroconvulsive threshold in rabbits even a week following their stay in complete darkness.

Even more important phenomena of supersensitivity and epileptization were discovered in fully or partly denervated cortical islets with intact pial blood supply (Echlin & Battista, 1963; Ingvar, 1955b; Sharpless & Halpern, 1962). The regularity of spontaneous convulsive discharges, their form, and the facility with which they could be evoked by electrical or pharmacological stimulation resembled the activity of an epileptic focus. The effect of neural isolation did not depend much on the area of isolation and was practically identical in various animals and in humans. It manifested itself spontaneously during the application of stimulation to denervated tissue, as well as during humoral stimulation of the brain. Clinicians know the effect well because epileptiform disturbances are a complication of lobotomy (Garcia-Austt, Iniguez, Sengundo, Migliaro, & Perez, 1954). That these phenomena are connected with the nonutilization of cells was shown in the experiments made by Sharpless and Halpern (1962), and later by Rutledge, Ranck, and Duncan (1967). They succeeded in preventing development of supersensitivity by subjecting the isolated cortex to daily electrical stimulation, replacing normal stimulation.

Sharpless (1963) attempted to compare pharmacological denervation with surgical denervation. Twenty-four hours after the completion of a course of narcotic injections that had lasted several days, an islet of the neocortex was subpially isolated. It appeared that the parameters of its electrical reactions were in all respects identical to those registered in the chronically isolated cortex. Narcotization of animals with barbiturates for a period ranging from 26 days to 3 weeks led to a lowering of the threshold of Metrazol seizures and spontaneous convulsions. Incidentally, denervated structures as well as epileptic foci are distinguished by increased sensitivity to pharmacological agents, and their activity can be reliably suppressed by barbiturates, opiates, and other sedatives that exert no noticeable effect on normal elements (Stavraky, 1961).

Myslobodsky (1965, 1973) used a sensory deprivation procedure to study the SN−LR complexes and to find out whether it would be possible to demonstrate their evolution into W−S. Rabbits were kept in darkness with their eyelids sewn closed from birth to the age of 1 month. At this time they were carried in a container to a half-darkened operating room, and electrodes were implanted using unidirectional light sources. In deprived animals, the VEP, especially the secondary SN−LR complex, was remarkably suppressed. A stable stress theta-rhythm was registered in the occipital and sensorimotor leads.

The stress theta-rhythm, which in rats and rabbits may be recorded from the cortex, is originally a hippocampal rhythm. It was defined by Green and Arduini (1954) as a hippocampal correlate of nondifferentiated arousal similar to neocortical desynchronization. It has already been mentioned that its development was always associated with suppression of sensory theta-rhythm and, correspondingly, the SAD and the secondary SN−LR complex of the VEP, which are correlates of the low arousal level. Further research showed that the stress theta-rhythm may be a correlate of more specific functions. For example, it is believed that it may be associated with mechanisms of the orienting reaction (Grastyán, Lissák, Madarasz, & Konhoffer, 1959), processes of planning and organization of locomotor activity (Vanderwolf, 1969), mechanisms of motivated behavior and reward (Bruner, 1967; Kramis & Routtenberg, 1969), and so on.

If we discount the view that the hippocampal theta-rhythm does not exist as a single entity but is a set of rhythms of varying natures, then we must admit that there is something common at the root of hippocampal synchronization in each individual case. According to some data, movement can be excluded from among the number of possible uniting mechanisms, for it turned out that immobility does not eliminate the theta rhythm. It was also revealed that the desynchronization of electrical activity of the hippocampus during movement may take place (Bennett, 1969) and the theta rhythm may be absent during feeding or drinking behavior, which inevitably requires the active participation of locomotion (Pond, Lidsky, Levine, & Schwartzbaum, 1970).

It seems just as futile to seek correlates of the activity of the reward system in the hippocampal theta-rhythm, for it is also activated during stimulation of the negative zones of the brain (Routtenberg & Kramis, 1968). Besides, during eating and drinking the hippocampal theta-rhythm was absent, even though it appeared when points that evoked similar food reactions were stimulated (Pond *et al.*, 1970).

This creates the impression that this rhythm may serve first of all as an indicator of the orienting reaction and moderate forms of defensive behavior. Even if sexual and food motivation evoke theta rhythm in the hippocampus, they do so only when their intensity grows extreme or is induced by tetanization of the hypothalamus. Apparently, hippocampal theta-rhythm appears in all cases when a stimulus is new or unexpected or is excessively intense, or when the situation becomes stressful. In that sense it was very clearly defined as a *stress rhythm* (Anochin, 1964).

The foregoing poses a question about the value of distinguishing between the hippocampal reaction to activation and neocortical arousal. To paraphrase that question teleologically, what are the advantages of synchronized arousal in the hippocampus if it also has a desynchronized type of arousal reaction at its disposal? It is well known that the activation reaction, especially the one that emerges from prolonged stimulation of the centers of negative reinforcement, evokes catastrophic consequences in the somatic status of the animal, which may be cured when the positive zone is stimulated (Lilly, 1960). It is also known that in its organization the stress rhythm may be considered a typical example of inhibitory synchronization, similar in some respects to identical rhythms in the thalamus and neocortex (Eccles, 1965).

Since one rhythm combines, as it were, both activation and inhibition, it is possible that stress rhythm serves as a sparing activator, a unique activating buffer that prevents the destructive action of powerful drive evoking fluxes of desynchronizing impulses. This is not contradicted by the emergence of a hippocampal theta-rhythm during stimulation of the reward system, since this electrical stimulation may evoke an activation of drive, and the feeling of reward is probably associated with the potentials of the off-effect. In this connection it is also not excluded that the stress rhythm, frequently developing in the process of self-stimulation, could be a nonspecific by-product emerging exclusively through the excitation of circuits leading to the mesencephalon and hippocampus.

Thus, in this experiment sensory deprivation led to the activation of stress rhythm as a correlate of behavioral arousal and stress (Melzack, 1965). Not only is it not a precursor of W–S-type discharges, but it even correlates with a decrease in the probability of their emergence.

If its appearance creates favorable conditions for seizure development we may be dealing with discharges of the hyperdepolarizing type, phenomena primarily associated with grand mal epilepsy. In rabbits X-irradiated in utero on the twenty-third day of prenatal development, stress rhythm was a constant phenomenon (Ivanitsky, 1966), and these rabbits displayed lowered thresholds and prolonged seizure afterdischarges to direct epicortical stimulation.

Perhaps, in general, the law of denervation is justified when used to explain focal seizures or grand mal fits. Indeed, if epileptiform rhythm develops in isolated nervous tissue, it relates mostly to electrographic episodes of a generalized grand mal seizure, an activity connected with hyperdepolarization of the elements. However, information given previously indicates that with few exceptions the problem of W–S complexes can hardly be studied on the basis of discharges of that type. Although epileptiform rhythms of different genesis frequently combine, these combinations have definite limits. Wave–spike complexes may evolve into a convulsive afterdischarge that, apparently, is explained by the excessive potentiation of synapses functioning in the recurrent activation circuits; but it never happens the other way around.

The difference between the two types of convulsive rhythmicity is probably linked not only with the specifics of the operating regimes of nervous nets, but also with the nature of mediation in the different groups of synapses. Barbiturates, which as we know efficiently control convulsive discharges of the hyperdepolarization type, predominantly suppress the activity of adrenergic, but not cholinergic, synapses, as shown by Johnson, Roberts, and Straughan (1969). At the same time W–S complexes, judging from the pharmacological sensitivities of their experimental models, are probably related to the functioning of the cholinergic system. The suppression by barbiturates of W–S discharges only takes place when a clear narcotic effect is also noted.

Sensory deprivation leads much more frequently to the organization of rhythmicity resembling W–S complexes (Parsons-Smith, 1953; Zislina & Novikova, 1971), but the mechanism of this phenomenon is just as unclear. It would be very arbitrary to predict any shifts that may take place when an afferent channel is eliminated in a system of neurons having a multitude of inputs of different quality, especially if it is one that normally blocks the passage of impulses to the given center. The particular and general consequences of desynaptization (disturbance of membrane permeability, structure of the elements, their afferents, systems of mediation, and so on) may be reduced to a common denominator only by the introduction of a multitude of assumptions, most of which have as yet not been proved experimentally.

A study of the role of supersensitivity to acetylcholine seemed promising. Convulsive poisons were shown to act far more intensely against an anticholinesterase background. In fact, such a background is in itself able to increase the probability of the emergence of convulsive afterdischarges, and even to evoke them (Echlin & Battista, 1963). This includes W–S discharges (Ivanitsky & Myslobodsky, 1965). I have already mentioned that in conditions of neuronal isolation the epileptogenic capability of acetylcholine increases somewhat so that no pretreatment of the cortex with anticholinesterase is needed to evoke hypersynchronous discharges.

Rosenberg and Echlin (1965) arrived at the conclusion that the main reason for the development of supersensitivity in isolated cortical islets is the increase in the permeability of the membranes to acetylcholine and a considerable decrease (50–60%) in the activity of acetylcholinesterase, emerging 6–10 months after surgery. Duncan, Rutledge, and Domino (1968) found that as a result of cortical undercutting acetylcholinesterase activity decreased by 24%. Hebb, Krnjević, and Siler (1963) used the histochemical method to demonstrate the decrease in the activity of cholinesterase and cholineacetylase in isolated cortex slabs.

A stable increase in the acetylcholine content of the brain by 40–60% was observed in some strains of mice. In these mice it was much simpler to evoke convulsive activity than in normal mice (Naruse, Kato, Kurokawa, Haba, &

Yabe, 1960). There are also data on the disturbance of the mediation of acetylcholine during the abstinence syndrome (Schuster, 1953) and sensory deprivation (Maletta & Timiras, 1967), both of which are accompanied by a lowering of seizure thresholds.

However, increases in convulsive readiness and in sensitivity to acetylcholine do not always correlate with one another. Analysis of the causes of the increase in convulsive readiness in a neuronally isolated cortical slab, recently made in the laboratories of Krnjević, Reiffenstein, and Silver (1970a,b) and Spehlman (1971), demonstrated that there was no supersensitivity to acetylcholine. Its ability to activate the cells during iontophoresis was negligible. This seems to indicate that sensitivity of neuronal elements to the mediator is not an inherent property, but only a consequence of cholinergic innervation; and it therefore disappears when the cholinergic fibres are damaged (Krnjević *et al.*, 1970a). This does not mean, however, that the development of supersensitivity to the mediator may not take place when its activity is for some reason lowered, even though the cholinergic input is intact. For the time being there is no possibility either to prove or to disprove that assumption. Further studies must be made of the sensitivity to acetylcholine of individual brain areas.

The effects of irradiation in the prenatal and early postnatal ontogenesis show that disturbance of the system of mediation may affect only individual structures of the brain stem or the basal ganglia.

However, the possibility is not to be excluded that during relatively normal sensitivity of a denervated center to acetylcholine a neuron, because of a purely anatomical reorganization of the neural circuits, may acquire the ability to activate a larger number of elements than normally. In the view of Krnjević *et al.* (1970b) supersensitivity is a possible result of the unbalancing of excitation and inhibition effects with a predominance, naturally, of the former. It was assumed that this is due to the destruction of the large pyramids and the relative predominance of the small ones, which apparently function in the circuits of recurrent activation (Takahashi, Kubota, & Uno, 1967).

In a neuronally isolated islet of immature neocortex an increase in the number of axon-collaterals (sprouting) was noticed, and this seemed a very likely reason for an increase in its excitability (Purpura & Housepian, 1961). This is another type of anatomical reorganization of neural circuits. It is possible that sprouting in some measure compensates for the disuse of synapses; we would expect a lowering of the islet excitability. In any case, in the presence of regular electrical stimulation of its surface one observes a normalization of the thresholds of convulsive afterdischarges (Rutledge, Duncan, & Beatty, 1969; Sharpless & Halpern, 1962) and of the activity of cholinesterase (Duncan *et al.*, 1968).

Rutledge *et al.* (1969) demonstrated that the number of axon-collaterals drops in the isolated cortex of a mature cat. Yet, if the surface of the isolated islet is regularly stimulated by electrical stimuli imitating synaptic activity, their number remains normal. I have presented data on an increase in convulsive readiness in animals raised in darkness and subjected to an enucleation operation. The pathohistological changes developed in them have been described sufficiently accurately, but no direct information was given on the presence of sprouting. On the contrary, they generally mentioned a decrease in dendritic branching of the pyramids, a decrease in the number of spines, and a decrease in the length and number of sprouts of the stellate cells (Globus & Scheibel, 1967; Valverde, 1967).

It is no less problematic whether pharmacological denervation, evoking practically the same phenomena as surgery, does so by way of sproutings. Thus, although in the spinal cord sprouting is known to be the cause of the maladaptive restoration of functions, this does not mean that supersensitivity in isolated cortex should be explained in the same way. It would seem that it could equally well be considered a desensitizing factor. However, it is probably still too early to exclude this process from consideration.

This is particularly relevant in cases of prenatal injuries, where the remaining nerve cells have greater possibilities of establishing new abnormal contacts than do mature deafferented neurons.

Embryonal injuries caused by radiation evoke other disturbances able to lead to the development of an epileptic syndrome. Among them, changes on the part of the dendrites call for particular attention. The direction in which their morphological reorganization will proceed can be imagined on the basis of the ideas of Cajal, used by Valverde (1967) to explain the atypical orientation of cell sprouts in denervated cortex. If we proceed from the assumption that regeneration develops according to the same laws as embryonal development, we should postulate identical changes also in irradiated cortex. Indeed, during maturing of the neocortex the increase in the number of synapses may result from the formation of new dendrites or the increase in the number of branches of the existing ones. Since to all intents and purposes the number of dendrites of the first order does not change in adults as compared with newborns (Schadé, 1959, cited according to Caveness *et al.,* 1968), it is thought that during denervation ramification of peripheral dendrites is obstructed. The resulting desynaptization, taking into account that the dendrites account for 80% of brain volume, is able to have catastrophic consequences. It has been shown that in an epileptic lesion created in the cortex of monkeys with alumna cream, there is a disappearance of cells, predominantly of the pyramids in the deep layers and small cells in the surface layers. In the remaining cells the dendrites were changed, the number of their branchings was smaller, and the number of spines decreased sharply (Westrum *et al.,* 1964). It will be noted that these changes closely resemble those caused by X-irradiation in utero (Berry *et al.,* 1963; Hicks & D'Amato, 1963).

6   Conclusions

The main question posed in this book is whether there exist precursors of abnormal W–S-type discharges. It may be answered in the positive. In animals this precursor is the secondary SN–LR complex, which is particularly well expressed in the visual cortex but can also be registered in other areas since it is a universal component of any evoked potential.

The SN–LR complex may also be determined as a representative and first component of the sensory discharge of the aftereffect (SAD). In its turn the SAD is an evoked fragment of the sensory theta-rhythm, i.e., the basic rhythm of a quiet waking rabbit or rat. It is particularly well expressed and often exalted in drive reduction situations and may therefore also be called the relaxation, reward, or pleasure rhythm. Thus, the sensory theta-rhythm or pleasure rhythm may be the precursor of hypersynchronous W–S type discharges.

The human brain has at its disposal more rigid mechanisms for the control of these forms of rhythmicity, but they are not always obvious. Studies of the reactivity of the human brain indicate that here, too, the same precursors of W–S discharges can be traced, but normally they are encountered only during a certain age period, a certain period of sleep, and, naturally, in cases where the control mechanisms of cerebral activity are already decompensated.

Experiments in animals and clinical studies strengthen the conviction that most of the specific conditions leading to the organization of W–S discharges are connected with a special type of abnormal activity, asthenia, or areactivity of the desynchronizing brain centers. In this connection it is preferable to speak of the centrasthenic genesis of petit mal epilepsy and W–S discharges, since the centrencephalic conception in its contemporary form presupposes more than certain anatomic limits for epileptogenous changes within the subcortical structures. It suggests a special type of activity in these centers that is able to induce an abnormal bisynchronous and generalized cortical rhythm. In this respect the terms centrencephalic and centrenergetic coincide, which is justified by neither experimental nor clinical–physiological data. Therefore the view of centrasthenic epilepsy reverses the sign of the presumed centrencephalon activity and does not oblige it to be the indispensable pacemaker of epileptiform rhythms.

Naturally, it is as yet unknown whether asthenia of the activating centers does not really mean a specific breakup or temporary disturbance of the whole system of control of neocortical activity, which manifests itself in the characteristic W–S rhythm and a lowering of the tonus of centers responsible for maintaining wakefulness. Such a breakup may be connected with endogenous (genetic or endocrine factors) and exogenous causes. An example of the latter are local W–S rhythms registered in the area of the lesion and, correspondingly, wave–spike forms in the evoked potentials, coexisting with the VEP of a normal configuration on the opposite side. In such cases centrasthenia may apparently play the role of an important additional condition, a maximum risk factor that facilitates the transition of interictal activity into the bed of generalized and bilaterally synchronized paroxysms. It is a factor that promotes the formation of focal activity into typical 3-per-second W–S discharges.

It may, however, turn out that there are also genuine autonomous forms of inhibitive hypersynchronization in addition to the centralized ones. For some reason focal W–S discharges, too, are conceived as initially such a form. It is tempting to connect them with disturbances of the system controlling neocortical rhythmicity directly at the level of the executive apparatus, i.e., the synaptic structures by means of which the centers of the limbic and reticular systems implement more generalized effects. Although this assumption is not the only possibility, there are grounds to suspect that diffuse pathology of this controlling system, about which we know very little as yet, is also the basis of bisynchronous W–S discharges. It is therefore useful to look not only for electrographic expressions and mechanisms of this central asthenia, but also for mechanisms of focal inhibitory hypersynchronization, taking into account that we may arrive at an understanding of the problem of petit mal epilepsy via an analysis of the focal W–S discharges.

Recognition of the equipotentiality of different brain structures in their ability to form local inhibitory hypersynchronous rhythms directly presupposes the polycentric principle of the organization of W–S pacemakers. Any centers of the hypnogenic system, especially the basal ganglia, preoptic area, and orbitofrontal cortex, may act as initiators of hypersynchronous discharges when cortical activity is released from the control of the limbic–reticular disinhibitory system.

Derangement of this system leads to elimination of interareal EEG difference and reduction of EEG frequency, perhaps due to release of some reticulocortical afferents that operate on cortical inhibitory interneurons.

Changes in EEG and evoked potentials in most *waking* patients strikingly resemble those of *sleeping* normal subjects. This phenomenon was interpreted as a *fragment* of sleep or a *partial sleep* of the cortex. We believe, as did Speransky (1932), that for petit mal epilepsy "the basic features of neural mechanisms of sleep and the epileptic fit are similar."

This assumption implies that a partial sleep background predisposes the brain to the development of petit mal. It is partially reflected by facilitation of W–S during lower arousal levels and initial stages of non-REM sleep and their suppression during a state of arousal and in REM sleep. It is believed that the lower activity of the right hemisphere in the waking state, with its ability to develop a greater amount of slow-wave patterns, especially in situations of reward, makes it more vulnerable to the petit mal epilepsy.

This study did not include consideration of all the implications of the theory for clinical use. It is clear, however, that in many cases a "merciful regime," as also excessive use of sedatives, will at the least promote a conservation of the conditions maintaining the epileptic process. Drive-inducing activities, we believe, are highly recommended for patients who have petit mal epilepsy.

True, when studying reactive potentials in some epileptics, cases were also found (it is not as yet clear whether they are specific forms or a stage in the development of the process), where in addition to the intensification of the inhibitory synaptic action in the cortex, there was also an abnormal intensification of the activity of excitatory processes; and this makes it tempting to connect this phenomenon with the activity of the recurrent excitatory circuits. Although this warning should be heeded in the preceding cases, apparently they require a more thoroughly balanced treatment, able to suppress absences and prevent an aggravation by seizures of the grand mal type. There are optimistic symptoms indicating that a study of evoked potentials will help to differentiate between such subtypes.

References

Adey, W. R. Organization of the rhinencephalon. In H. H. Jasper (Ed.), *Reticular formation of the brain.* Boston: Little, Brown, 1958. P. 621.

Airapetianz, M. G. *Derangement of higher nervous activity after prenatal X-irradiation.* Moscow: Nauka, 1966.

Ajmone-Marsan, C. The thalamus. Data on its functional anatomy and some aspects of thalamo-cortical integration. *Arch. Ital. Biol.,* 1965, **103,** 847.

Akert, K., & Andersson, B. Experementeller beitrag zur physiologie des nucleus caudatus. *Acta Physiol. Scand.,* 1951, **22,** 261.

Alexandrovskaya, M. M. Some morphological changes of the central nervous system in white rat x-irradiated in utero. *Med. Radiol.,* 1959, **4,** 79.

Alexandrovskaya, M. M. Comparative morphological studies of the brain changes in rats x-irradiated with 50, 150 and 200 r on the 12th day of embriogeny. *Ann. of the Institute of Higher Nervous Activity, Pathophysiol. Series,* 1962, **10,** 125.

Andermann, F. Absence attacks and diffuse neuronal disease. *Neurology,* 1967, **17,** 205.

Andermann, K., Berman, S., Cooke, P. M., Dickson, J., Gastaut, H., Kennedy, A., Margerison, J., Pond, D. A., Tizard, J. P. M., & Walsh, E. G. Self-induced epilepsy. *Arch. Neurol.,* 1962, **6,** 49.

Andersen, P., & Andersson, S. A. *Physiological basis of alpha-rhythm.* New York: Appleton, 1968.

Angeleri, F., Ferro-Milone, F., & Parigi, S. Electrical activity and reactivity of the rhinencephalic, pararhinencephalic and thalamic structures: Prolonged implantation of electrodes in man. *EEG. Clin. Neurophysiol.,* 1964, **16,** 100.

Anochin, P. K. Neurophysiological basis of electrocortical activity of the brain. In *Contemporary problems of electrophysiological investigations of the central nervous system.* Moscow: Medizina, 1964. P. 132.

Artiuchina, N. I. Morphological characteristics of structural changes in the central nervous system during postnatal development of white X-irradiated in utero. In *2nd*

Conference on the influences of ionizing radiation on the central nervous system. Abstracts of papers, 1958. P. 10.

Arushanian, E. B., & Belozertsev, Yu. A. Inhibitory effects of caudate nucleus on the electrical activity of somatosensory neurons. *Fiziol. Journal,* 1970, **56**, 1111.

Bancaud, J., Talairach, J., Bonis, A., Szikla, G., Morel, P., & Bordsferrer, M. *La stereoencéphalographie dans l'epilepsie.* Paris: Masson, 1965.

Bancaud, J., Talairach, J., Morel, P., Bresson, M., Bonis, A., Geier, S., Hemon, E., & Buser, P. "Generalized" epileptic seizures elicited by electrical stimulation of the frontal lobe in man. *EEG Clin. Neurophysiol.,* 1974, **37**, 275.

Bartley, S. H. Central mechanisms of vision. In *Handbook of physiology. Neurophysiology I.* Washington, D.C.: American Physiological Society, 1959. P. 713.

Batsel, H. L. Electroencephalographic synchronization and desynchronization in the chronic "cerveau isole" of the dog. *EEG Clin. Neurophysiol.,* 1960, **12**, 421.

Bennett, T. L. Evidence against the theory that hippocampal theta is a correlate of voluntary movement. *Commun. Behav. Biol.,* 1969, **4**, 165.

Bergamasco, B. Excitability cycle of the visual cortex in normal subjects during psychosensory rest and cardiovascular activation. *Brain Res.,* 1966, **2**, 51.

Bergamini, L., & Bergamasco, B. Possibility of the clinical use of the sensory evoked potentials transcranially recorded in man. *EEG Clin. Neurophysiol.,* Suppl., 1967, **26**, 114.

Bergonie, J., & Tribandeau, L. In A. A. Manina, *Radiational lesions and repair processes in the ontogeny of mammal central nervous system.* Moscow: Medizina, 1964.

Berlyne, D. E. The reward-value of indifferent stimulation. In J. T. Tapp (Ed.), *Reinforcement and behavior.* New York: Academic Press, 1969. P.178.

Berry, M., Clendinnen, B. G., & Ears, J. T. Electrocortical activity in the rat x-irradiated during early development. *EEG Clin. Neurophysiol.,* 1963, **15**, 91.

Bickford, R. G., Daly, D., & Keith, H. Convulsive effect of light stimulation in children. *Amer. J. Dis. Child.,* 1953, **86**, 170.

Bickford, R. G., & Klass, D. W. Sensory precipitation and reflex mechanisms. In H. H. Jasper, A. A. Ward, Jr., & A. Pope (Eds.), *Basic mechanisms of epilepsies.* Boston: Little, Brown, 1969. P.543.

Bignall, K. E., Imbert, M., & Buser, P. Optic projections to non-visual cortex of the cat. *J. Neurophysiol.,* 1966, **29**, 396.

Bigum, H. B., Dustman, R. E., & Beck, E. C. Visual and somatosensory evoked responses from mongoloid and normal children. *EEG Clin. Neurophysiol.,* 1970, **28**, 576.

Black, S. L., & Vanderwolf, C. H. Thumping behavior in rabbit. *Physiol. and Behavior,* 1969, **4**, 445.

Bogacz, J., St. Laurent, J., & Olds, J. Dissociation of self-stimulation and epileptiform activity. *EEG Clin. Neurophysiol.,* 1965, **19**, 75.

Bogen, J. E., & Bogen, G. M. The other side of the brain. III. The corpus callosum and creativity. *Bull. L.A. Neurol. Sci.,* 1969, **34**, 141.

Bradley, P. B. The central action of certain drugs in relation to the reticular formation of the brain. In H. H. Jasper (Ed.), *Reticular formation of the brain.* Boston: Little, Brown, 1958. P.123.

Broughton, R., Meier-Ewert, K. H., & Ebe, M. Evoked visual, somato-sensory and retinal potentials in photosensitive epilepsy. *EEG Clin. Neurophysiol.,* 1969, **27**, 373.

Broughton, R., Poire, R., & Tassinari, C. A. The electrodermogram (Tarchenoff effect) during sleep. *EEG Clin. Neurophysiol.,* 1965, **18**, 691.

Bruner, A. Self-stimulation in the rabbit: An anatomical map of stimulation effects. *J. Compar. Neurol.,* 1967, **131**, 615.

Buchbaum, M., & Fedio, P. Hemispheric differences in evoked potentials to verbal and nonverbal stimuli in the left and right visual fields. *Physiol. and Behavior,* 1970, 5, 207.

Buchthal, F., & Lennox, M. The EEG effect of Metrazol and photic stimulation in 682 normal subjects. *EEG Clin. Neurophysiol.,* 1953, 5, 545.

Buchwald, N. A., Hull, C. D., & Trachtenberg, M. C. Concomitant behavioral and neural inhibition and disinhibition in response to subcortical stimulation. *Exper. Brain Res.,* 1967, 4, 58.

Bureau, M., Guey, J., Dravet, C., & Roger, J. A study of the distribution of petit mal absences in the child in relation to his activities. *EEG Clin. Neurophysiol.,* 1968, 25, 513.

Burke, W., & Sefton, A. J. Discharge patterns of principal cells and interneurones in lateral geniculate nucleus of rat. *J. Physiol.,* 1966, 187, 202. (a)

Burke, W., & Sefton, A. J. Recovery of responsiveness of cells of lateral geniculate nucleus of rat. *J. Physiol.,* 1966, 187, 213. (b)

Burke, W., & Sefton, A. J. Inhibitory mechanisms in lateral geniculate nucleus of rat. *J. Physiol.,* 1966, 187, 231. (c)

Butler, S. R., & Glass, A. Asymmetries in the electroencephalogram associated with cerebral dominance. *EEG Clin. Neurophysiol.,* 1974, 36, 481.

Cadilhac, J., & Passouant, P. Influence of various phases of night sleep on the epileptic discharges in man. *EEG Clin. Neurophysiol.,* 1964, 17, 441.

Caggiula, A. R. Analysis of the copulation-reward properties of posterior hypothalamic stimulation in male rats. *J. Comp. and Physiol. Psychol.,* 1970, 70, 339.

Cajal, S. R. Y. *Studies on the cerebral cortex.* London: Lloyd-Luke, 1955.

Cannon, W. B., & Rosenblueth, A. *The supersensitivity of denervated structures.* New York: Macmillan, 1949.

Caveness, W. F., Carsten, A. L., Roizin, L., & Schade, J. P. Pathogenesis of x-irradiation effects in the monkey cerebral cortex. *Brain Res.,* 1968, 7, 1.

Cernacek, J., & Ciganek, L. The cortical electroencephalographic response to light stimulation in epilepsy. *Epilepsia,* 1962, 3, 303.

Cesa-Bianchi, M. G., Mancia, M., & Mutani, R. Experimental epilepsy induced by cobalt powder in lower brain stem and thalamic structures. *EEG Clin. Neurophysiol.,* 1967, 22, 525.

Charlton, M. H., & Yahr, M. D. Long-term follow-up patients with petit mal. *Arch. Neurol.,* 1967, 16, 595.

Chatrian, G. E., Somasundaram, M., & Tassinari, C. A. DC changes recorded transcranially during "typical" three per second spike and wave discharges in man. *Epilepsia,* 1968, 9, 185.

Chernishevskaya, I. A. Morphological changes in the rabbit brain, x-irradiated in the later period of prenatal development. *Ann. of the Institute of Higher Nervous Activity. Pathophysiol. Series,* 1962, 10, 138.

Christophe, J., & Rémond, A. Dyssynergia cerebellaris myoclonica de Ramsay hunt. Etude clinique et électroencéphalographique. *Revue Neurologique,* 1951, 84, 256.

Churchill, J. A. The relationship of epilepsy to breech delivery. *EEG Clin. Neurophysiol.,* 1959, 11, 1.

Cigánek, L. The EEG response (evoked potential) to light stimulus in man. *EEG Clin. Neurophysiol.,* 1961, 13, 165.

Cigánek, L. Excitability cycle of the visual cortex in man. *Ann. N.Y. Acad. Sci.,* 1964, 112, 241.

Cigánek, L. A comparative study of visual, auditory and somatosensory EEG responses in man. *Exper. Brain Res.,* 1967, 4, 118.

Clemente, C. D. Forebrain mechanisms related to internal inhibition and sleep. *Conditional Reflexes,* 1968, **3**, 145.

Clemente, C. D., Sterman, M. B., & Wyrwicka, W. Post-reinforcement EEG synchronization during alimentary behavior. *EEG Clin. Neurophysiol.,* 1964, **16**, 335.

Cohn, R. The effect of strychninization of certain massa intermedia nuclei in cats. *EEG Clin. Neurophysiol.,* 1949, **1**, 520.

Cohn, R. Rhythmic after-activity in visual evoked responses. *Ann. N.Y. Acad. Sci.,* 1964, **112**, 281.

Cohn, R. A neuropathological study of a case of petit mal epilepsy. *EEG Clin. Neurophysiol.,* 1968, **24**, 282.

Cooke, J. P., Brown, S. O., & Krise, G. M. Prenatal chronic gamma irradiation and audiogenic seizures in rats. *Exper. Neurol.,* 1964, **9**, 243.

Cooper, R. M., & Taylor, L. H. Thalamic reticular system and central grey: Self-stimulation. *Science,* 1967, **156**, 102.

Cornill, L., & Gastaut, H. Etude electroencephalographique de la dominance sensorielle d'un hemisphere cerebral. *Presse Medicale,* 1947, **37**, 421.

Courtois, A., & Cordeau, J. O. Changes in cortical responsiveness during transition from sleep to wakefulness. *Brain Res.,* 1969, **14**, 199.

Crain, S. M. Development of "Organotypic" bioelectric activities in central nervous tissues during maturation in culture. *Internat. Rev. Neurobiol.,* 1966, **9**, 1.

Creutzfeldt, O. D., & Kuhnt, U. The visual evoked potential: Physiological, developmental and clinical aspects. *EEG Clin. Neurophysiol.,* Suppl., 1967, **26**, 29.

Creutzfeldt, O. D., & Struck, G. Neurophysiology and morphology of the chronically isolated cortical islet in the cat: Brain potential and neuron activity of an isolated nerve cell population without afferent fibers. *Arch. Psychiat. Nervenkr.,* 1962, **203**, 708.

Crosby, E. C., Humphrey, T., & Lauer, R. *Correlative anatomy of the nervous system.* New York: Macmillan, 1962.

Dahl, E., Gjerstad, L. I., & Skrede, K. K. Persistent thalamic and cortical barbiturate spindle activity after ablation of the orbital cortex in cat. *EEG Clin. Neurophysiol.,* 1972, **33**, 485.

Davis, H., Davis, P. A., Loomis, A. L., Harvey, E. N., & Hobart, G. Human brain potentials during the onset of sleep. *J. Neurophysiol.,* 1938, **1**, 24.

Dawson, G. D. Cerebral responses to electrical stimulation of peripheral nerve in man. *J. Neurol. Neurosurg. Psychiatry,* 1947, **10**, 137.

Delgado, J. M. R. *Physical control of the mind.* New York: Harper, 1969.

Demetrescu, M., & Julien, R. M. Local anesthesia and experimental epilepsy. *Epilepsia,* 1974, **15**, 235.

Dewan, E. M. Occipital alpha rhythm, eye position and lens accommodation. *Nature,* 1967, **214**, 975.

Doti, R. W. General discussion. In H. H. Jasper (Ed.), *Reticular formation of the brain.* Boston: Little, Brown, 1958, P.582.

Duncan, J. A., Rutledge, L. T., & Domino, E. F. Acetylcholinesterase activity in partially isolated cerebral cortex after prolonged intermittent stimulation. *Exp. Neurol.,* 1968, **20**, 268.

Dustman, R. E., & Beck, E. C. Phase of alpha brain waves, reaction time and visually evoked potentials. *EEG Clin. Neurophysiol.,* 1965, **18**, 433.

Ebe, M., Mikami, T., & Ito, E. Cortical evoked potentials by photic stimulation at various adaptation levels of retina in man. *Tohoku J. Exp. Med.,* 1963, **80**, 9.

Eccles, J. C. Inhibition in thalamic and cortical neurones and its role in phasing neuronal discharges. *Epilepsia,* 1965, **6**, 89.

Echlin, F. A., & Battista, A. Epileptiform seizures from chronic isolated cortex. *Arch. Neurol.,* 1963, 9, 154.

Ekiert, H., & Bigo, B. The value of chlorpromazine as activating EEG method in cases of epilepsy. *EEG Clin. Neurophysiol.,* 1959, 11, 177.

Elian, M. EEG, epilepsy and precocious puberty. *EEG Clin. Neurophysiol.,* 1970, **28**, 642.

Fabisch, W., & Darbyshire, R. Report on an unusual case of self-induced epilepsy with comments on some psychological and therapeutic aspects. *Epilepsia,* 1965, 6, 335.

Farber, D. A. *The functional maturation of the brain in early stages of ontogenesis.* Moscow: Prosveschenie Publ. House, 1969.

Feeney, D. M., & Gullotta, F. P. Suppression of seizure discharges and sleep spindles by lesion of the rostral thalamus. *Brain Res.,* 1972, 45, 254.

Fifkova, E., & Marsala, J. In J. Bures, M. Petran, & J. Zachar (Eds.), *Electrophysiological methods in biological research.* New York: Academic Press, 1967. P.653.

Fisher, R. Catography of inner space. In R. K. Siegel & L. J. West (Eds.), *Hallucinations. Behavior, experience, and theory.* New York: Wiley, 1975. P.197.

Fois, A., Rosenberg, C., & Gibbs, F. A. The electroencephalogram in phenylpyruvic oligophrenia. *EEG Clin. Neurophysiol.,* 1955, 7, 569.

Fridman, B. O. EEG role in the evaluation of the state of compensation of epilepsy in childhood. In *Problems of the children's psychiatry.* Leningrad: Medgiz, 1961. Vol. 25, P.129.

Friesen, G. Roentgenomorphoses in drosophila. *Biol. Zurn.,* 1935, 4, 36.

Fuster, B. EEG activation under natural or induced sleep. *EEG Clin. Neurophysiol.,* Suppl., 1953, 4, 108.

Fuster, J. M., Creutzfeldt, O. D., & Straschill, M. Intracellular recording of neuronal activity in the visual system. *Z. Vergl. Physiol.,* 1965, 49, 605.

Gainotti, G. Emotional behavior and hemispheric side of the lesion. *Cortex,* 1972, 8, 41.

Garcia-Austt, Jr., E., Iniguez, R. A., Sengundo, J. P., Migliaro, E., & Perez, L. A. Epileptic activity in isolated cortical areas in man. *EEG Clin. Neurophysiol.,* 1954, 6, 536.

Gastaut, H. Clinical and electroencephalographic correlates of generalized spike and wave bursts occurring spontaneously in man. *Epilepsia,* 1968, 9, 179.

Gastaut, H., & Hunter, J. An experimental study of the mechanism of photic activation in idiopathic epilepsy. *EEG Clin. Neurophysiol.,* 1950, 2, 263.

Geets, W. Influence possible de l'irradiation prénatale sure le développement de l'activité électrique cérébrale chez l'home. *Acta Neurol. Belg.,* 1968, 68, 654.

Geinisman, Y., & Myslobodsky, M. S. Rate of maturation and peculiarity of derangement of the visual cortex in rabbits x-irradiated in the middle and end of embriogeny. In I. Piontkovsky (Ed.), *Studies in neuroradioembriological effect.* Moscow: Nauka, 1966. P.88.

Gellhorn, E., & Loofborrow, G. N. *Emotions and emotional disorders. A neurophysiological study.* New York: Harper, 1963.

Gibberd, F. B. The clinical features of petit mal. *Acta Neurol. Scand.,* 1966, 42, 176.

Gibbs, F. A., Davis, H., & Lennox, W. G. The electro-encephalogram in epilepsy and in conditions of impaired consciousness. *Arch. Neurol. Psychiat.,* 1935, 34, 1133.

Gibbs, E. L., & Gibbs, F. A. Diagnostic and localizing value of electroencephalographic studies in sleep. *Res. Publ. Assoc, Res. Nerv. and Ment. Dis.,* 1947, **26**, 366.

Gibbs, F. A., & Gibbs, E. L. *Atlas of electroencephalography.* Reading, Massachusetts: Addison-Wesley, 1952.

Gibson, J. G., & Kennedy, W. A. A clinical EEG study in a case of obsessional neurosis. *EEG Clin. Neurophysiol.,* 1960, **12**, 198.

Glasser, G. H., & Hoefer, F. A. Electroencephalographic changes during and after encephalitis. *EEG Clin. Neurophysiol.,* 1950, **2**, 361.

Globus, A., & Scheibel, A. B. Synaptic loci on visual cortical neurons of the specific afferent radiation. *Exp. Neurol.,* 1967, **18**, 116.

Gloor, P. Generalized cortico-reticular epilepsies. Some considerations on the pathophysiology of generalized bilaterally synchronous spike and wave discharges. *Epilepsia,* 1968, **9**, 249.

Gloor, P. Generalized spike and wave discharges: A consideration of cortical and subcortical mechanisms of their genesis and synchronization. In H. Petsche & M. A. B. Brazier (Eds.), *Synchronization of EEG activity in epilepsies.* New York: Springer-Verlag, 1972. P.382.

Goldring, S. The role of prefrontal cortex in grand mal convulsions. *Arch. Neurol.,* 1972, **26**, 109.

Golla, F., Graham, S., & Walter, W. G. The electroencephalogram in epilepsy. *J. Ment. Sci.,* 1937, **83**, 137.

Gowers, W. R. *Epilepsy and other chronic convulsive diseases.* New York: Dover, 1885.

Grastyán, E., Lissák, K., Madarasz, I., & Konhoffer, H. Hippocampal electrical activity during the development of conditioned reflexes. *EEG Clin. Neurophysiol.,* 1959, **11**, 409.

Green, J. B. Seizures on closing the eyes. *Neurology,* 1968, **18**, 391.

Green, J. B. Photosensitive epilepsy—the electro-retinogram and visually evoked response. *Arch. Neurol.,* 1969, **20**, 191.

Green, J. B., & Aroduini, A. A. Hippocampal electrical activity in arousal. *J. Neurophysiol.,* 1954, **17**, 532.

Groth, H., Weled, B., & Batkin, S. A. A comparison of monocular visually evoked potentials in human neonates and adults. *EEG Clin. Neurophysiol.,* 1970, **28**, 478.

Guerrero-Figueroa, R., Barros, A., de Balbian Vebster, F., & Heath, R. G. Experimental "petit mal" in kittens. *Arch. Neurol.,* 1963, **9**, 297. (a)

Guerrero-Figueroa, R., Barros, A., de Balbian Vebster, F., & Heath, R. G. Some inhibitory effects of attentive factors on experimental epilepsy. *Epilepsia,* 1963, **4**, 225. (b)

Guselnicov, V. I., & Supin, A. Ya. *Rhythmical activity of the brain.* Moscow: Moscow Univ. Press, 1968.

Hackett, J. T., & Marzynski, T. J. Positive reinforcement and visual evoked potentials in cat. *Brain Res.,* 1971, **26**, 57.

Halliday, A. M. The electrophysiological study of myoclonus in men. *Brain,* 1967, **90**, 241.

Halpern, M. Effects of midbrain central gray matter lesions on escape avoidance behavior in rats. *Physiol. Behavior,* 1968, **3**, 171.

Hassler, R., & Dieckmann, G. Arrest reaction, delayed inhibition and unusual gaze behavior resulting from stimulation of the putamen in awake, unrestrained cats. *Brain Res.,* 1967, **5**, 504.

Hayne, R. A., Belinson, L., & Gibbs, F. A. Electrical activity of subcortical areas in epilepsy. *EEG Clin. Neurophysiol.,* 1949, **1**, 437.

Heath, R. G. *Studies in schizophrenia: A multidisciplinary approach to mind—brain relationships.* Cambridge, Massachusetts: Harvard Univ. Press, 1954.

Hebb, C. O., Krnjević, K., & Siler, A. Effect of under cutting on the acetylcholinesterase and choline acetyltransferase activity in cats' cerebral cortex. *Nature,* 1963, **198**, 692.

Hecaen, H., & Angeleriques, R. *Le cécité psychique.* Paris: Masson, 1963.

Herberg, L. J., Tress, K. H., & Blundell, J. E. Raising the threshold in experimental epilepsy by hypothalamic and septal stimulation and by audiogenic seizures. *Brain,* 1969, **92**, 313.

Hess, R., Scollo-Lavizzari, G., & Wyss, F. E. Borderline cases of petit mal status. *European Neurol.,* 1971, **5,** 137.

Hicks, S. P. Some aspects of developmental neurology: A review. *Cancer Res.,* 1957, **17,** 251.

Hicks, S. P. Radiation as an experimental tool in mammalian developmental neurology. *Physiol. Rev.,* 1958, **38,** 337.

Hicks, S. P., & D'Amato, C. J. Low dose radiation of the developing brain. *Science,* 1963, **141,** 903.

Hill, D. EEG in episodic psychotic and psychopathic behavior. A classification of data. *EEG Clin. Neurophysiol.,* 1952, **4,** 419.

Hishikawa, Y., Yamamoto, J., Furuya, E., Yamada, Y., Miyazaki, K., & Kaneko, Z. Photosensitive epilepsy: Relationships between the visual evoked responses and the epileptiform discharges induced by intermittent photic stimulation. *EEG Clin. Neurophysiol.,* 1967, **23,** 320.

Hodos, W., & Valenstein, E. S. Motivational variables affecting the rate of behavior maintained by intracranial stimulation. *J. Compar. Physiol. Psychol.,* 1960, **53,** 502.

Hoebel, B. G. Inhibition and disinhibition of self-stimulation and feeding. Hypothalamic control and postingestional factors. *J. Compar. Physiol. Psychol.,* 1962, **66,** 89.

Hoening, J., & Hamilton, C. M. Epilepsy and sexual orgasm. *Acta Psychiat. Scand.,* 1960, **35,** 448.

Holowach, J., Thunston, D. L., & O'Leary, J. L. Petit mal epilepsy. *Pediatrica,* 1962, **30,** 893.

Howell, D. A. Unusual centrencephalic seizure patterns. *Brain,* 1955, **78,** 199.

Hubel, D. H., & Nauta, W. J. H. Electrocorticograms of cats with chronic lesions of the nostral mesencephalic segmentum. *Federat. Proc.,* 1960, **19,** 287.

Hull, C. D., Buchwald, N. A., & Vieth, J. Cortical intracellular analysis of responses to inhibitory and disinhibitory stimuli. *Brain Res.,* 1967, **6,** 12.

Humphrey, D. R. Re-analysis of the antidromic cortical response. II. On the contribution of cell discharge and PSPs to the evoked potentials. *EEG Clin. Neurophysiol.,* 1968, **25,** 421.

Humphrey, M. E., & Zangwill, O. L. Cessation of dreaming after brain injury. *J. Neurol., Neurosurg. & Psychiat.,* 1951, **14,** 322.

Hunter, J., & Jasper, H. H. Effects of thalamic stimulation in unanaesthetised animals. *EEG Clin. Neurophysiol.,* 1949, **1,** 305.

Idelson, A. V. Cited by Lomov, B. F. Manual interaction in the process of tactile perception. In A. Leontyev, A. Luriya, & A. Smirnov (Eds.), *Psychological research in the USSR.* Moscow: Progress Publishers, 1966. P.267.

Ingvar, D. H. Reproduction of the 3-per-second spike and wave EEG pattern by subcortical electrical stimulation in cats. *Acta Physiol. Scand.,* 1955, **33,** 137. (a)

Ingvar, D. H. Electrical activity of isolated cortex of the unanesthetized cat with intact brainstem. *Acta Physiol. Scand.,* 1955, **33,** 151. (b)

Ingvar, D. H. Cortical state of excitability and cortical circulation. In H. H. Jasper (Ed.), *Reticular formation of the brain.* Boston: Little, Brown, 1958. P.381.

Ito, M. Excitability of medial forebrain bundle neurons during self-stimulation behavior. *J. Neurophysiol.,* 1972, **35,** 652.

Ivanitsky, A. M. Interrelation between the function, development and the structure of cortical structure in ontogeny. Cand. Sci. Dissertation, Moscow, 1955.

Ivanitsky, A. M. *Neurophysiological analysis of inborn brain derangements.* Moscow: Nauka, 1966.

Ivanitsky, A. M., & Myslobodsky, M. S. On the secondary response of the visual cortex in rabbits. *Z. Viss. Nerv. Deijat.*, 1965, **15**, 887.

Jasper, H. H. Electrical signs of epileptic discharge. *EEG Clin. Neurophysiol.*, 1949, **1**, 11.

Jasper, H. H., & Droogleever-Fortuyn, J. Experimental studies of the functional anatomy of petit mal epilepsy. *Res. Publ. Assoc, Res. Nerv. and Ment. Dis.*, 1947, **26**, 272.

Jasper, H. H., & Kershman, J. Electroencephalographic classification of the epilepsies. *Arch. Neurol.*, 1941, **45**, 903.

Johnson, E. S., Roberts, M. H. T., & Straughan, D. W. The responses of cortical neurones to monoamines under differing anaesthetic conditions. *J. Physiol.*, 1969, **203**, 261.

Katsuhito, A., & Powell, E. W. Differential projections of habenular nuclei. *J. Compar. Neurol.*, 1968, **132**, 263.

Kiloh, L. G., & Osselton, J. M. *Clinical electroencephalography.* London: Butterworths, 1966.

Kimeldorf, D. J., & Hunt, E. G. *Ionizing radiation. Neural function and behavior.* New York: Academic Press, 1965.

Kimura, D. Multiple response of the visual cortex of the rat to photic stimulation. *EEG Clin. Neurophysiol.*, 1962, **14**, 115.

Kimura, D. Left-right differences in the perception of melodies. *Quart. J. Exp. Psychol.*, 1964, **14**, 355.

Klingberg, F., Pickenhain, I., & Neumeister, K. The effect of a single intrauterine x-irradiation on the postnatal development of the higher nervous activity and the electrocortico-gram of rats. *Acta Biol. Med. German,* 1967, **19**, 503.

Kok, E., *Visual agnosias.* Leningrad: Medizina, 1967.

Kolomeitseva, I. A., & Myslobodsky, M. S. The role of embrionic brain damage in the organisation of epileptiform activity in adult animals. *Z. Pathophysiol.*, 1969, **6**, 11.

Kondrat'eva, I. N. On inhibition in neuronal system of visual area. *Z. Viss. Nerv. Deijat.*, 1964, **14**, 1069.

Kondrat'eva, I. N. Cyclic changes in cortical neuronal activity after brief stimuli. In V. S. Rusinow (Ed.), *Electrophysiology of the central nervous system.* New York: Plenum, 1970. P.239.

König, J. F. R., & Klippel, R. A. *The rat brain: A stereotaxic atlas of the forebrain and lower parts of the brainstem.* Baltimore: Williams and Wilkins, 1963.

Konnikov, B. A. On the problem of the positive reinforcement areas: Self-stimulation of the lateral geniculate body. *SSSR Physiol. Zurn.*, 1974, **60**, 1777.

Kooi, K. A., & Bagchi, B. K. Visual evoked responses in man. Normative data. *Ann. N.Y. Acad. Sci.*, 1964, **112**, 254.

Kooi, K. A., Eckman, H. G., & Thomas, M. H. Observations on the response to photic stimulation in organic cerebral dysfunction. *EEG Clin. Neurophysiol.*, 1957, **9**, 239.

Kooi, K. A., Thomas, M. H., & Mortenson, F. N. Photoconvulsive and photomyoclonic responses in adults. An appraisal of their clinical significance. *Neurology,* 1960, **10**, 1051.

Kopeloff, N., Whittier, J. R., Pacella, B. L., & Kopeloff, L. M. The epileptogenic effect of subcortical alumina cream in the rhesus monkey. *EEG Clin. Neurophysiol.*, 1950, **2**, 163.

Kramis, R. C., & Routtenberg. A. Rewarding brain stimulation, hippocampal activity, and footstamping in the gerbil. *Physiol. Behavior,* 1969, **4**, 7.

Krnjević, K., Randić, M., & Straughan, D. W. Cortical inhibition. *Nature,* 1964, **201**, 1294.

Krnjević, K., Reiffenstein, R. J., & Silver, A. Chemical sensitivity of neurons in long isolated slabs of cat cerebral cortex. *EEG Clin. Neurophysiol.*, 1970, **29**, 269. (a)

Krnjević, K., Reiffenstein, R. J., & Silver, A. Inhibition and paroxysmal activity in long isolated cortical slabs. *EEG Clin. Neurophysiol.*, 1970, **29**, 283. (b)

Kruglikov, R. I. *Some peculiarities of higher nervous functions x-irradiated in the prenatal period of life.* Thesis Cand. Dissertation. Moscow, 1961.

Kruglova, L. I., & Rubinova, F. S. *Social and labour rehabilitation of epileptic patients.* Leningrad: Medgiz Publishing House, 1968.

Kudinova, M. P., & Myslobodsky, M. S. Peculiarities of alpha-afterdischarges of the visual evoked responses in man. *Z. Viss. Nerv. Deijat.*, 1970, **20**, 85.

Laget, P., & Humbert, R. Facteurs influensant la résponse electroencéphalographique à la photostimulation chez l'enfant. *EEG Clin. Neurophysiol.*, 1954, **6**, 591.

Lange, H. de. Relationship between critical flicker-frequency and a set of low frequency characteristics of the eye. *J. Opt. Soc. Amer.*, 1954, **44**, 380.

Lennox, M. *Epilepsy and related disorders.* Boston: Little, Brown, 1960.

Lerique-Koechlin, A., Nekhorocheff, M., & Le Mansec, M. Valeur diagnostique de la stimulation lumineuse intermittente chez l'enfant. *Revue Neurologique,* 1950, **82**, 575.

Levin, P., Wyss, F. E., Scollo-Lavizzari, G., & Mess, R. Evolution of seizure patterns in experimental epilepsy. *European Neurology,* 1968, **1**, 65.

Lewis, E. G., Dustman, R. E., & Beck, E. C. The effect of alcohol on visual and somatosensory evoked responses. *EEG Clin. Neurophysiol.*, 1970, **28**, 202.

Li, C. L., & Chou, S. N. Cortical intracellular synaptic potentials and direct cortical stimulation. *J. Cell. Comp. Physiol.*, 1962, **60**, 1.

Lilly, J. C. Learning motivated by subcortical stimulation. The "start" and "stop" patterns of behavior. In E. R. Ramey & D. S. O'Doherty (Eds.), *Electrical studies of unanesthetized brain.* New York: Harper, 1960. P.78.

Lilly, J. C., & Shurley, J. T. Experiments on solitude in maximum achievable physical isolation with water suspension of intact healthy persons. In B. E. Flaherty (Ed.), *Psychophysiological aspects of space flight.* New York: Columbia Univ. Press, 1961. P.238.

Lindsley, D. B. Bilateral differences in brain potentials from the two cerebral hemispheres in relation to laterality and stuttering. *J. Exp. Psychol.*, 1940, **26**, 211.

Lindsley, D. B. Basic perceptual processes and the EEG. *Psychiatric Research Reports,* 1956, **6**, 161.

Lindsley, D. B. The reticular activating system and perceptual integration. In D. Sheer (Ed.), *Electrical stimulation of the brain.* Austin: Texas Univ. Press, 1961. P.331.

Lindsley, D. B., Bowden, J., & Magoun, H. W. Effect upon the EEG of acute injury to brain stem activating system. *EEG Clin. Neurophysiol.*, 1949, **1**, 475.

Lippold, O. *The origin of the alpha rhythm.* London: Churchill Livingston, 1973.

Livanov, M. N. Curves of electrical reactivity of the brain cortex in animals and in man in normal state and in pathology. *Izv. AN SSSR, Seria Biol.*, 1944, **6**, 332.

Livanov, M. N. Concerning the establishment of temporary connections. *EEG Clin. Neurophysiol.*, Suppl., 1960, **13**, 185.

Livanov, M. N. *Some problems of ionizing radiation action on the nervous system.* Moscow: Medgiz Publishing House, 1962.

Livanov, M. N., & Preobrazenskaya, N. S. Curves of electrical reactivity of the cerebral cortex in response to light stimulation of increasing brightness in brain-wounded patients. *Probl. Fiziol. Opt.*, 1947, **4**, 96.

Livingston, S., Torres, I., Pauli, L. L., & Rider, R. V. Petit mal epilepsy. Results of prolonged follow-up study of 117 patients. *JAMA*, 1965, **194**, 227.

Lomov, B. F. Manual interaction in the process of tactile perception. In A. Leontyev, A.

Luriya, & A. Smirnov (Eds.), *Psychological research in the USSR.* Moscow: Progress Publishers, 1966. P.267.

Lorente de No, R. Architechtonics and structure of the cerebral cortex. In J. F. Fulton (Ed.), *Physiology of the nervous system.* London: Oxford University Press, 1943.

Lucking, C. H. Visual evoked potentials in epilepsy. *EEG Clin. Neurophysiol.,* 1969, 27, 628.

Lundervold, A., Henriksen, G. F., & Fegersten, L. The spike and wave complex: A clinical correlation. *EEG Clin. Neurophysiol.,* 1959, 11, 13.

Luria, A. R. *The human brain and psychical processes.* Moscow, 1970.

Madsen, J. A., & Bray, P. F. The coincidence of diffuse electroencephalographic spike–wave paroxysms and brain tumors. *Neurology,* 1966, 16, 546.

Maletta, G. J., & Timiras, P. S. Acetyl and butyryl-cholinesterase activity of selected brain areas in developing rats after neonatal x-irradiation. *J. Neurochem.,* 1966, 13, 75.

Maletta, G. J., & Timiras, P. S. Acetylcholinesterase activity in optic structures after complete light deprivation from birth. *Exp. Neurol.,* 1967, 19, 513.

Maekawa, K., & Purpura, D. P. Intracellular study of lemniscal and non-specific synaptic interactions in thalamic ventrobasal neurons. *Brain Res.,* 1967, 4, 308.

Manina, A. A. *Radiational lesions and repair processes in the ontogeny of mammal central nervous system.* Moscow: Medizina, 1964.

Marco, L. A., & Brown, T. S. Thalamic inhibitory interneurone. *Nature,* 1966, 211, 1388.

Marcus, E. M., & Watson, C. W. Bilateral synchonous spike waves electrographic patterns in the cat. *Arch. Neurol.,* 1966, 14, 601.

Matsumoto, H., & Ajmone-Marsan, C. Cortical cellular phenomena in experimental epilepsy: Interictal manifestations. *Exp. Neurol.,* 1964, 9, 286. (a)

Matsumoto, H., & Ajmone-Marsan. C. Cortical cellular phenomena in experimental epilepsy: Ictal manifestations. *Exp. Neurol.,* 1964, 9, 305. (b)

Maulsby, R. L. An illustration of emotionally evoked theta rhythm in infancy: Hedonic hypersynchrony. *EEG Clin. Neurophysiol.,* 1971, 31, 157.

McDonald, D. A., & Potter, J. M. The distribution of blood to the brain. *J. Physiol.,* 1951, 114, 356.

Melnitchuk, P. V. *Clinico-electrophysiological analysis of reactivity measures in epilepsy.* Unpublished doctoral thesis, Moscow, 1971.

Melsen, S. The value of photic stimulation in the diagnosis of epilepsy. *J. Nerv. Ment. Dis.,* 1958, 128, 508.

Melzack, R. Effects of early experience on behavior: Experimental and conceptual considerations. In P. H. Hock & J. Zubin (Eds.), *Psychopathology of perception.* New York: Grune, Stratton, Vol. 20, 271, 1965.

Metrakos, K., & Metrakos, J. D. Is the centrencephalic EEG inherited as a dominant? *EEG Clin. Neurophysiol.,* 1961, 13, 289.

Milhorat, T. H., Baldwin, M., & Hantman, D. A. Experimental epilepsy after rostral reticular formation excision. *J. Neurosurg.,* 1966, 24, 595.

Miller, D. S. Effects of low-level radiation on audiogenic convulsive seizures in mice. In T. J. Haley & R. S. Snider (Eds.), *Response of the nervous system to ionizing radiation.* New York: Academic Press, 1962. P.513.

Miller, N. E. Learning and performance motivated by direct stimulation of the brain. In D. E. Sheer (Ed.), *Electrical stimulation of the brain.* Austin: Univ. of Texas Press, 1961, P.387.

Mirsky, A. F., Bloch-Rojas, S., & McNarry, W. F. Experimental "petit mal" epilepsy produced with chlorambucil. *Acta Biol. Exp. (Warsc.),* 1966, 26, 55.

Morgan, A. H., McDonald, J., & MacDonald, H. Differences in bilateral alpha activity as a function of experimental task, with a note on lateral eye movement and hypnotizability. *Neuropsychologia,* 1971, 9, 459.

Morgane, P. J. The function of limbic and rhinic forebrain—limbic system and reticular formation in the regulation of food and water intake. *Ann. N.Y. Acad. Sci.,* 1969, **157,** 806.

Morocutti, C., Sommer-Smith, J. A., & Creutzfeldt, O. D. Das visuelle reaktions-potential bei normalen versuchs personen und charakteristische veränderungen bei epileptikern. *Arch. Psychiatrie Nervenkr.,* 1966, **208,** 234.

Morrell, F., & Baker, L. Effects of drugs on secondary epileptogenic lesions. *Neurology,* 1961, **11,** 651.

Morrell, L. K., & Salamy, J. S. Hemispheric asymmetry of electrocortical responses to speech stimuli. *Science,* 1971, **174,** 164.

Moruzzi, G., & Magoun, H. W. Brain stem reticular formation and activation of the EEG. *EEG Clin. Neurophysiol.,* 1949, **1,** 455.

Mosovich, A., & Tallaferro, A. Studies on EEG and sex function orgasm. *Disease Nerv. System,* 1954, **15,** 218.

Mulholland, T. B., & Evans, C. R. Ocubomota functions and the alpha activation cycle. *Nature,* 1966, **211,** 1278.

Mundy-Castle, A. C. An analysis of central responses to photic stimulation in normal adults. *EEG Clin. Neurophysiol.,* 1953, **5,** 1.

Myslobodsky, M. S. The characteristics of the primary response to light in ontogeny of rabbits x-irradiated in utero. *Dokladi Academi Nauk,* 1964, **159,** 690.

Myslobodsky, M. S. *Peculiarities of the visual evoked potentials in ontogeny of rabbits x-irradiated in utero.* Thesis of Cand. Sci. dissertation, Moscow, Institute of Higher Nervous Activity & Neurophysiology, USSR Academy of Sci., 1965.

Myslobodsky, M. S. The part played by secondary evoked potentials in the organization of the driving response in the visual cortex in rabbit. *Z. Viss. Nervn. Deijat.,* 1966, **16,** 303.

Myslobodsky, M. S. Nature of wave-spike discharges: Centrencephalic or centrasthenic? *Z. Viss. Nervn. Deijat.,* 1968, **18,** 850. (a)

Myslobodsky, M. S. Transformation of visual evoked potential in the rabbit into a discharge of wave-spike type. *Z. Viss. Nervn. Deijat.,* 1968, **18,** 660. (b)

Myslobodsky, M. S. *Formation of hypersynchronous activity of the cerebral cortex in animal and in man.* Thesis of D. Sci. dissertation, Moscow, 1970. (a)

Myslobodsky, M. S. On the probable mechanism of functioning of pleasure system. *Z. Viss. Nervn. Deijat.,* 1970, **20,** 1298. (b)

Myslobodsky, M. S. Some implications of the abnormal excitability cycle. *Z. Viss. Nervn. Deijat.,* 1970, **20,** 602. (c)

Myslobodsky, M. S. Neurophysiological mechanisms of photogenic epilepsy. *Uspehi Sovremen. Physiolog.,* 1971, **2,** 91.

Myslobodsky, M. S. Cyclical changes of excitability of the visual cortex in epileptic patients. *Z. Nervrpat. Psychiatr.,* 1972, **72,** 886.

Myslobodsky, M. S. Two forms of asymmetry of the averaged evoked potentials of the cerebral hemispheres in man. *Z. Viss. Nervn. Deijat.,* 1973, **23,** 979.

Myslobodsky, M. S., & Fridrandsky, A. I. Averaged evoked potentials in epileptic patients. *Z. Neuropathol. Psychiatr. (Korsakov),* 1971, **8,** 1132.

Myslobodsky, M. S., & Kuznetsova, G. D. Photic self-stimulation in rat. *Dokladi Akademii Nauk SSSR,* 1971, **198,** 978.

Naquet, R., Denavit, M., Lanoir, J., & Albe-Fessard, D. Temporary or definitive alterations of diencephalic zones in cat: Their relationship with EEG cortical activity and sleep. *EEG Clin. Neurophysiol.,* 1964, **17,** 448.

Naruse, H., Kato, M., Kurokawa, M., Haba, R., & Yabe, T. Metabolic defects in a convulsive strain of mouse. *J. Neurochem.*, 1960, **5**, 359.

Nauta, W. J. H. Some neural pathways related to the limbic system. In E. R. Ramey & D. S. O'Doherty (Eds.), *Electrical studies of the unanesthetized brain.* New York: Harper, 1960. P.1.

Nauta, W. J. H., & Whitlock, D. C. An anatomical analysis of the non-specific thalamic projection system. In J. F. Delafresnaye (Ed.), *Brain mechanisms and consciousness.* Oxford: Blackwell, 1954. P.81.

Nebes, R. D. Superiority of the minor hemisphere in commisurotomized man for the perception of part-whole relations. *Cortex,* 1971, **7**, 333.

Newman, B. L., & Feldman, S. M. Electrophysiological activity accompanying intracranial self-stimulation. *J. Compar. Physiol. Psycho.*, 1964, **57**, 244.

Niedermeyer, E. Sleep electroencephalograms in petit mal. *Arch. Neurol.*, 1965, **12**, 625.

Niedermeyer, E. Generalized seizure discharges and possible precipitative mechanisms. *Epilepsia,* 1966, **7**, 23.

Niedermeyer, E. *The generalized epilepsies. A clinical electroencephalographic study.* Springfield, Illinois: C. C. Thomas, 1972.

Niedermeyer, E., Laws, E. R., & Walker, A. E. Depth EEG findings in epileptics with generalized spike–wave complexes. *Arch. Neurol.*, 1969, **21**, 51.

Nielson, H. C., & McIver, A. H. Cold stress and habenular lesion effects on rat behaviors. *J. Appl. Physiol.*, 1966, **21**, 655.

Novikova, L. A. *Electrical activity of the brain after the derangement of distant receptors.* Doctoral dissertation, Moscow, 1965.

Ohtani, T., Hirano, T., & Kita, Y. Sexual excitement as a form of epileptic attacks. *J. Kyoto Prefect. Med. Univ.*, 1962, **71**, 759.

Okujava, V. M. *Basic neurophysiological mechanisms of epileptic activity.* Tbilisi: Ganatleba Publishing House, 1969.

Olds, J. Differentiation of reward system in the brain by self-stimulation techniques. In E. R. Ramey & D. S. O'Doherty (Eds.), *Electrical studies of unanesthetized brain.* New York: P.B. Hoeber, 1960. P.17.

O'Leary, J. Discussion. In V. B. Mountcastle (Ed.), *Interhemispheric relation and cerebral dominance.* Baltimore: Johns Hopkins Univ. Press, 1967. P.39.

Parsons-Smith, G. Activity of the cerebral cortex in amblyophia. *Brit. J. Ophthalmol.*, 1953, **37**, 359.

Patarnello, L. Sexual orgasm and epilepsy. Clinical and electroencephalographic considerations of a case. *Arch, Psicol. Neurol. Psichiat.*, 1963, **24**, 558.

Patry, G., Lyagoubi, S., & Tassinari, C. A. Subclinical "electrical status epilepticus" induced by sleep in children. *Arch. Neurol.*, 1971, **24**, 242.

Peacock, S. M., Jr. Averaged "after-activity" and the alpha-regeneration cycle. *EEG Clin. Neurophysiol.*, 1970, **28**, 287.

Penfield, W. Epilepsy, neurophysiology, and some brain mechanisms related to consciousness. In H. H. Jasper & A. Pope (Eds.), *Basic mechanisms of epilepsies.* Boston: Little, Brown, 1969. P.791.

Penfield, W., & Erickson, T. C. *Epilepsy and the functional anatomy of the human brain.* Springfield, Illinois: C. C. Thomas, 1941.

Penfield, W., & Jasper, H. *Epilepsy and the functional anatomy of the human brain.* Boston: Little, Brown, 1954.

Perot, P. Cited in Jasper, H., Mechanisms of propagation: Extracellular studies. In H. Jasper, A. Ward, & A. Pope (Eds.), *Basic mechanisms of the epilepsies.* Boston: Little, Brown, 1969. P.421.

Petuchov, V. V. *Electrophysiological analysis of the evoked and spontaneous activity of "spike–wave" type in cat.* Unpublished Candidate sci. thesis, Moscow, 1968.

Piontkovsky, I. A. *Function and structure of the brain in animals x-irradiated in antenatal period.* Moscow: Nauka, 1964.

Pollack, I. Selected developments in psychophysics, with implications for sensory organization. In W. A. Rosenblith (Ed.), *Sensory communication.* Cambridge, Massachusetts: MIT Press, 1961. P.89.

Pollen, D. A. Intracellular studies of cortical neurons during thalamic induced wave and spike. *EEG Clin. Neurophysiol.,* 1964, **17,** 398.

Pollen, D. A., & Ajmone-Marsan, C. Cortical inhibitory postsynaptic potentials and strychninization. *J. Neurophysiol.,* 1965, **28,** 342.

Pollen, D. A., & Lux, H. D. Conductance changes during inhibitory postsynaptic potentials in normal and strychninized cortical neurons. *J. Neurophysiol.,* 1966, **29,** 3699.

Pollen, D. A., Perot, P., & Reid, K. H. Experimental bilateral wave and spike from thalamic stimulation in relation to level of arousal. *EEG Clin. Neurophysiol.,* 1963, **15,** 1017.

Pollen, D. A., Reid, K. H., & Perot, P. Microelectrode studies of experimental 3/sec wave and spike in the cat. *EEG Clin. Neurophysiol.,* 1964, **17,** 57.

Pollen, D. A. & Sie, P. G. Analysis of thalamic induced wave and spike by modifications in cortical excitability. *EEG Clin. Neurophysiol.,* 1964, **17,** 154.

Polyanski, V. B. Relationships between rapid and slow activity in the response of the visual cortex of alert rabbits to rhythmic photic stimulation. *Z. Viss. Nervn. Deijat.,* 1966, **16,** 298.

Pond, F. J., Lidsky, T. I., Levine, M. S., & Schwartzbaum, J. S. Hippocampal electrical activity during hypothalamic-evoked consummatory behavior in rats. *Psychonomic Science,* 1970, **21,** 21.

Porter, R. W., & Bors, E. Modulation of brain stem electrical activity by visceral (urinary bladder) distension. *EEG Clin. Neurophysiol.,* 1962, **14,** 527.

Porter, R. W., Cavanaugh, E. G., Critchlow, B. V., & Sawyer, C. H. Localized changes in electrical activity of the hypothalamus in estrous cats following vaginal stimulation. *Amer. J. Physiol.,* 1957, **189,** 145.

Powell, T. P. S., & Cowan, W. M. The connexions of the midline and intralaminar nuclei of the thalamus of the rat. *J. Anat.,* 1954, **88,** 307.

Preobrazenskaya, E. S. Phenomena of irritation of the visual lobe due to its traumatic lesion. *Neuropathol., Psychiatr.,* 1945, **14,** 38.

Prince, D. A. The depolarization shift in 'epileptic' neurons. *Exp. Neurol.,* 1968, **21,** 467. (a)

Prince, D. A. Inhibition in 'epileptic' neurons. *Exp. Neurol.,* 1968, **21,** 307. (b)

Proctor, F., Prince, D. A., & Morrel, F. Primary and secondary spike foci following depth lesions. *Arch. Neurol.,* 1966, **15,** 151.

Purpura, D. P., & Cohen, B. Intracellular recording from thalamic neurons during recruiting responses. *J. Neurophysiol.,* 1962, **25,** 621.

Purpura, D. P., & Housepian, E. M. Morphological and physiological properties of chronically isolated immature neocortex. *Exp. Neurol.,* 1961, **4,** 377.

Purpura, D. P., McMurtry, J. G., & Malkawa, K. Synaptic events in ventrolateral thalamic neurons during suppression of recruiting responses by brain stem reticular stimulation. *Brain Res.,* 1966, **1,** 63.

Purpura, D. P., & Shofer, R. J. Cortical intracellular potentials during augmenting and recruiting responses. I. Effects of injected hyperpolarizing currents on evoked membrane potential changes. *J. Neurophysiol.,* 1964, **27,** 117.

Purpura, D. P., & Shofer, R. J. Modification of ontogenetic patterns in mammalian brain. In E. A. Asratyan (Ed.), *Progress in Brain Research,* 1968, **22,** 458.

Ralston, B., & Ajmone-Marsan, C. Thalamic control of certain normal and abnormal cortical rhythms. *EEG Clin Neurophysiol.*, 1956, **8**, 559.

Rhodes, L. E., Dustman, R. E., & Beck, E. C. The visual evoked response: A comparison of bright and dull children. *EEG Clin. Neurophysiol.*, 1969, **27**, 364.

Robertson, R. T., & Lynch, G. S. Orbito-frontal modulation of EEG spindles. *Brain Res.*, 1971, **28**, 562.

Rogina, V., & Serafetinides, E. A. Epilepsy and behavior disorders in patients with generalized spike and wave complexes. *EEG Clin. Neurophysiol.*, 1962, **14**, 376.

Roitbak, A. I. Electrical phenomena in the cortex during the extinction of orienting and conditioned reflex. *EEG Clin. Neurophysiol., Suppl.*, 1960, **13**, 91.

Rosenberg, P., & Echlin, F. A. Cholinesterase activity of chronic partially isolated cortex. *Neurology*, 1965, **15**, 700.

Rosenblum, I. Light deprivation as a means of lowering electroshock thresholds in rabbits. *Exp. Neurol.*, 1963, **8**, 30.

Ross, J. J., Johnson, L. C., & Walter, R. D. Spike and wave discharges during stages of sleep. *Arch. Neurol.*, 1966, **14**, 399.

Rossi, G. F., & Rosadini, G. Experimental analysis of cerebral dominance in man. In C. H. Milliken & I. Darley (Eds.), *Brain mechanisms underlying speech and language*. New York: Grune and Stratton, 1967. P.167.

Routtenberg, A., & Kramis, R. C. Hippocampal correlates of aversive midbrain stimulation. *Science*, 1968, **160**, 1363.

Rutledge, L. T., Duncan, J. A., & Beatty, N. A study of pyramidal cell axon collaterals in intact and partially isolated adult cerebral cortex. *Brain Res.*, 1969, **16**, 15.

Rutledge, L. T., Ranck, J. B., & Duncan, J. A. Prevention of supersensitivity in partially isolated cerebral cortex. *EEG Clin. Neurophysiol.*, 1967, **23**, 256.

Sal y Rosas, F. El Comienzo de la epilepsia en las diferentes horas del dia. *Rev. Neuropsiquiat.*, 1952, **15**, 260.

Satterberg, J. A., & Ganz, L. Electroencephalographic and unit discharge patterns of the striate cortex of visual deprived kittens to photic stimuli. *EEG Clin. Neurophysiol.*, 1967, **23**, 91.

Sawa, M., Maruyama, N., & Kaji, S. Intracellular potential during electrically induced seizures. *EEG Clin. Neurophysiol.*, 1963, **15**, 209.

Sawyer, C. H. Reproductive behavior. In H. W. Magoun (Ed.), *Handbook of physiology. Section 1. Neurophysiology*. Baltimore, Maryland: Williams and Wilkins, 1960.

Sawyer, C. H., & Kawakami, M. Characteristics of behavioral and electroencephalographic afteractions to copulation and vaginal stimulation in the female rabbit. *Endocrinology*, 1959, **65**, 622.

Schade, J. P. Cited according to W. F. Caveness, A. L. Carsten, L. Roizin, & Schade, J. P. Pathogenesis of x-irradiation effects in the monkey cerebral cortex. *Brain Res.*, 1968, **7**, 1.

Schaper, B. Photic stimulation. *EEG Clin. Neurophysiol.*, 1957, **9**, 357.

Schefer, D. G., & Fuks, L. I. Changes of bioelectrical activity of the brain during hypothalamic epilepsy. *Zurn. Nevropathol., Psychiatr.*, 1969, **69**, 548.

Scheibel, M. E. & Scheibel, A. B. Structural organisation of nonspecific thalamic nuclei and their projection toward cortex. *Brain Research*, 1967, **6**, 60.

Schlag, J. Reactions and interactions to stimulation of the motor cortex of the cat. *J. Neurophysiol.*, 1966, **29**, 44.

Schlag, J. Discussion. In J. E. Skinner, & D. B. Lindsley, Electrophysiological and behavioral effects of blockade of the non-specific thalamo-cortical system. *Brain Res.*, 1967, **6**, 95.

Schuster, D. B. The EEG in sedative withdrawal. A case report. *EEG Clin. Neurophysiol.,* 1953, **5,** 607.

Schwartz, M., & Shagass, C. Recovery functions of human somatosensory and visual evoked potentials. *Ann. N.Y. Acad. Sci.,* 1964, **112,** 510.

Scollo-Lavizzari, G., & Hess, R. Sensory precipitation of epileptic seizures. Report on two unusual cases. *Epilepsia,* 1967, **8,** 157.

Sellden, U., & Hambert, O. Studies concerning the value of photic stimulation in different types of epilepsy. *EEG Clin. Neurophysiol.,* 1968, **24,** 87.

Sem-Jacobsen, C. W., & Torkildsen, A. Depth recording and electrical stimulation in the human brain. In E. R. Ramey & D. S. O'Doherty (Eds.), *Electrical studies of the unanesthetized brain.* New York: Hoeber, 1960. P.275.

Semmes, J., Weinstein, S., Gheht, L., & Teuber, H. L. *Somatosensory changes after penetrating brain wounds in man.* Vol. I. Cambridge, Massachusetts: Harvard Univ. Press, 1960.

Sepp, E. K., Zuker, M. B., & Shmidt, M. B. *Handbook of neurology.* Moscow: Medgiz, 1947.

Sharpless, S. K. Experimental studies of chronically isolated cortex. *EEG Clin. Neurophysiol.,* 1963, **15,** 1050.

Sharpless, S. K. Reorganization of function in the nervous system-use and disuse. *Annual Rev. Physiol.,* 1964, **26,** 357.

Sharpless, S. K., & Halpern, L. M. The electrical excitability of chronically isolated cortex studied by means of permanently implanted electrodes. *EEG Clin. Neurophysiol.,* 1962, **14,** 244.

Shearer, D. E., Flemming, D. E., Bigler, E. D., & Wilson, C. E. Suppression of photically evoked after-discharge bursting following administration of anticonvulsants in waking rats. *Pharmacol. Biochem. & Behav.,* 1974, **2,** 839.

Sheffield, F. D. A drive-reduction theory of reinforcement. In R. N. Haber (Ed.), *Current research in motivation.* New York: Holt, 1966. P.98.

Shelburne, S. A., Jr. Visual evoked responses to word and nonsense syllable stimuli. *EEG Clin. Neurophysiol.,* 1972, **32,** 17.

Shute, C. C. D., & Lewis, P. R. The ascending cholinergic reticular system: Neocortical olfactory and subcortical projections. *Brain,* 1967, **90,** 497.

Simonov, P. V. *Theory of reflection and psychophysiology of emotion.* Moscow: Nauka, 1970.

Skinner, J. E., & Lindsley, D. B. Electrophysiological and behavioral effects of blockade of the non-specific thalamo-cortical system. *Brain Res.,* 1967, **6,** 95.

Skrebitsky, V. G. Inhibition of inhibitory postsynaptic components of the visual evoked potentials during auditory stimulus presentation. *Z. Viss. Nervn. Deijat.,* 1967, **17,** 158.

Skrebitsky, V. G., & Voronin, L. L. Intracellular study of the activity of the visual cortex cells in unanesthetized rabbit. *Z. Viss. Nervn. Deijat.,* 1966, **16,** 864.

Skultety, F. M. The behavioral effects of destructive lesions of the periaqueductal gray matter in adult cats. *J. Compara. Neurol.,* 1958, **110,** 337.

Spehlman, R. Acetylcholine and the epileptiform activity in chronically isolated cortex. *Arch. Neurol.,* 1971, **24,** 495.

Spencer, W. A., & Kandel, E. R. Hippocampal neuron responses to selective activation of recurrent collaterals of hippocampofugal axons. *Exp. Neurol.,* 1961, **4,** 149.

Speransky, A. D. *Epileptic fit.* Moscow-Leningrad, 1932.

Sperry, R. W. Some general aspects of interhemispheric integration. In V. B. Mountcastle (Ed.), *Interhemispheric relations and cerebral dominance.* Baltimore, Maryland: Johns Hopkins Press, 1962. P.43.

Spiegel, E. A., Wycis, H. T., & Reyes, V. Diencephalic mechanisms in petit mal epilepsy. *EEG Clin. Neurophysiol.,* 1951, **3,** 473.

Spong, P., Haider, M., & Lindsley, D. B. Selective attentiveness and cortical evoked responses to visual and auditory stimuli. *Science,* 1964, **148,** 395.

Starzl, T. E., Niemer, W. T., Dell, M., & Forgrave, P. R. Cortical and subcortical electrical activity in experimental seizures induced by metrazol. *J. Neuropath. Exp. Neurol.,* 1953, **12,** 262.

Staunton, H. P., & Sasaki, K. Recruiting responses not dependent on orbitofrontal cortex. *Brain Res.,* 1971, **30,** 415.

Stavraky, C. W. *Supersensitivity following lesions of the nervous system.* Toronto: Univ. Press, 1961.

Stefanis, C., & Jasper, H. H. Recurrent collateral inhibition in pyramidal tract. *J. Neurophysiol.,* 1964, **27,** 855.

Stefanis, C., & Jasper, H. H. Strychnine reversal of inhibitory potentials in pyramidal tract neurones. *Internat. J. Neuropharmacol.,* 1965, **4,** 125.

Stevens, J. R. Central and peripheral factors in epileptic discharge. *Arch. Neurol.,* 1962, **7,** 330.

Stevens, J. R., Nakamura, Y., Milstein, V., Okuma, P., & Llinas, R. Central and peripheral factors in epileptic discharge. *Arch. Neurol.,* 1964, **11,** 463.

Stewart, L. F., & Dreifuss, F. E. "Centrencephalic" seizure discharges in focal hemispheral lesions. *Arch. Neurol.,* 1967, **17,** 60.

Stockard, C. R. Developmental rate and structural expression: An experimental study of twins, "double monsters" and single deformities, and the interaction among embrionic organs during their origin and development. *Amer. J. Anat.,* 1921, **28,** 115.

Straw, R. N., & Mitchell, C. L. A study on the duration of cortical after-discharge in the cat. *EEG Clin. Neurophysiol.,* 1966, **21,** 54.

Strobos, R. J., & Kavallinis, G. P. Changes in repeat electroencephalograms in epileptics. *Neurology,* 1968, **18,** 622.

Stutz, R. M., Butcher, R. E., & Rossi, R. Stimulus properties of reinforcing brain shock. *Science,* 1969, **163,** 1081.

Sudakov, K. V. On the interrelation of hypothalamus, midbrain reticular formation and thalamus in the mechanism of selective cortical activation in the state of hunger. *Fiziol. Journ. SSSR.,* 1965, **51,** 449.

Sutin, J., & Michael, R. P. Changes in brain electrical activity following vaginal stimulation in estrous and anestrous cats. *Physiol. Behavior,* 1970, **5,** 1043.

Svetlov, P. G., & Korsakova, G. F. Pathogenic influence of X-rays on rat embryogeny. In *Influence of ionizing radiation on the pregnancy, fetus and newborn.* Moscow: Medgiz, 1960.

Takahashi, K., Kubota, D., & Uno, M. Recurrent facilitation in cat pyramidal tract cells. *J. Neurophysiol.,* 1967, **30,** 22.

Taylor, D. C., & Ounsted, C. Biological mechanisms influencing the outcome of seizures in response to fever. *Epilepsia,* 1971, **12,** 33.

Temkin, O. *The falling sickness.* Baltimore, Maryland: Johns Hopkins Press, 1945.

Terzian, H. Behavioral and EEG effects of intracarotid sodium amital injections. *Acta Neurochirurg.,* 1964, **12,** 230.

Tonkova-Yampolsky, R. V. Cited in P. V. Simonov, Physiology of emotions and the theory of conditioned reflexes. In *Handbook of physiology. Physiology of higher nervous activity.* Part II. Moscow: Nauka, 1971. P.97.

Traugott, N. N., Kaidanova, S., & Meerson, Ja. Syndromes of parietal lobes lesions. In A. S.

Batuev (Ed.), *Evolution of functions of the parietal lobes of the brain.* Leningrad: Nauka, 1973. P.118.

Troupin, A. S. Photic activation and experimental data concerning colored stimuli. *Neurology,* 1966, **16**, 269.

Uchtomsky, A. A. *Lectures.* Leningrad: Leningrad University Press, 1938.

Ulett, G. A., & Johnson, L. C. Pattern, stability and correlates of photic electroencephalographic activation. *J. Nerv. Ment. Dis.,* 1958, **126**, 153.

Valenstein, E. S. Behavior elicited by hypothalamic stimulation. A prepotency hypothesis. *Brain Behav. Evol.,* 1969, **2**, 295.

Valenstein, E. S., & Valenstein, T. Interaction of positive and negative reinforcing neural systems. *Science,* 1964, **145**, 1456.

Valverde, F. Apical dendritic spines of the visual-cortex and light deprivation in the mouse. *Exp. Brain Res.,* 1967, **3**, 337.

Vanderwolf, C. H. Hippocampal electrical activity and voluntary movement in the rat. *EEG Clin. Neurophysiol.,* 1969, **26**, 407.

Van Reeth, P. C. A case of self-induced temporal lobe epilepsy and the problem of hedonic cerebral autostimulation. *Acta Neurol. Belg.,* 1959, **59**, 490.

Van Straaten, J. J. Relation between the secondary optic fibre system and the centrencephalic system. Localisation of a subcortical pacemaker for convulsions. *Arch. Internat. Physiol. Biochem.,* 1962, **70**, 483.

Varga, M. E., Kuznetsova, G. D., & Myslobodsky, M. S. A method of classical conditioning of washing reflex in rat. *Z. Viss. Nervn. Deijat.,* 1970, **20**, 719. (a)

Varga, M. E., Kuznetsova, G. D., & Myslobodsky, M. S. Changes of sensory afterdischarges to light during classical defensive conditioning in rats. *Z. Viss. Nervn. Deijat.,* 1970, **20**, 975. (b)

Varga, M. E., Kuznetsova, G. D., & Myslobodsky, M. S. Hypersynchronous afterdischarges and conditioned reflex in rats. *Z. Viss. Nervn, Deijat.,* 1971, **21**, 69.

Velasco, M., & Lindsley, D. B. Role of orbital cortex in regulation of the thalamo-cortical electrical activity. *Science,* 1965, **149**, 1375.

Velasco, M., Skinner, J. E., Asaro, K. D., & Lindsley, D. B. Thalamo-cortical system regulating spindle bursts and recruiting responses. I. Effect of cortical ablation. *EEG Clin. Neurophysiol.,* 1968, **25**, 464.

Vella, E. J., Butler, J. R., & Glass, A. Electrical correlate of right hemisphere function. *Nature. New Biology,* 1972, **236**, 125.

Vernandakis, A., & Timiras, P. S. Effects of whole body X-irradiation on electroshock seizure responses in developing rats. *Amer. J. Physiol.,* 1963, **205**, 177.

Vernandakis, A., Curry, J. J., Maletta, G. J., Irving, G., & Timiras, P. S. Convulsive responses in prenatally irradiated rats. *Experimental Neurol.,* 1966, **16**, 57.

Vidart, L., & Geier, S. Enregistrements teleencephalographiques chez des sujets epileptiques pendant le travail. *Rev. Neurol.,* 1967, **117**, 475.

Villablanca, J. The electrocorticogram in the chronic cerveau isole cat. *EEG Clin. Neurophysiol.,* 1965, **19**, 576.

Villablanca, J., Schlag, J., & Marcus, R. Blocking of experimental spike and wave by a localized forebrain lesion. *Epilepsia,* 1970, **11**, 163.

Walker, A. E., & Marshall, C. Stimulation and recording in man. In D. E. Sheer (Ed.), *Electrical stimulation of the brain.* Austin: Univ. of Texas Press, 1961. P.498.

Walker, A. E., & Marshall, C. The contribution of depth recording to clinical medicine. *EEG Clin. Neurophysiol.,* 1964, **16**, 88.

Walter, W. G., Dovey, V. J., & Shipton, H. Analysis of the electrical response of the human cortex to photic stimulation. *Nature,* 1946, **158,** 540.

Ward, A. A., Jr. Epilepsy. *Int. Rev. Neurobiol.,* 1961, **3,** 137.

Watanabe, S., Konishi, M., & Creutzfeldt, O. D. Postsynaptic potentials in the cat's visual cortex following electrical sitmulation of afferent pathways. *Exp. Brain Res.,* 1966, **1,** 272.

Watson, C. W., & Bowker, R. Effective parameters of photic stimulation for evocation of cerebral electrical abnormalities in man. *EEG Clin. Neurophysiol.,* 1965, **18,** 205.

Weinmann, H., Heyde, G., & Creutzfeldt, O. D. Development and pathological disturbances of the cortical visual evoked potential in children. *EEG Clin. Neurophysiol.,* 1966, **20,** 277.

Weir, B. Spike waves from stimulation of reticular core. *Arch. Neurol.,* 1964, **11,** 209.

Weir, B., & Sie, P. G. Extracellular unit activity in cat cortex during the spike-wave complex. *Epilepsia,* 1966, **7,** 30.

Werboff, J., Den Broeder, J., Havlena, J., & Sikov, M. R. Effects of prenatal X-ray irradiation on audiogenic seizures in the rat. *Exp. Neurol.,* 1961, **4,** 189.

Westrum, L. E., White, L. E., & Ward, A. A. Morphological studies of epileptic foci. *J. Neurosurg.,* 1964, **21,** 1033.

Wycis, H. T., Lee, A. J., & Spiegel, E. A. Simultaneous records on thalamic and cortical (scalp) potentials in schizophrenics and epileptics. *Confin. Neurol.,* 1949, **9,** 264.

Zammarchi, E., Luti, C., & Salvatori, Q. Petit mal and electroencephalographic changes found during sleep. *Rev. Clin. Pediatr.,* 1967, **79,** 128.

Zemskaya, A. G. *Focal epilepsy in childhood.* Leningrad: Medizina, 1971.

Zislina, N. N., & Novikova, L. A. The influence of visual deafferentation on spontaneous and evoked neuronal activity of the rabbit visual cortex. *Z. Viss. Nervn. Deijat.,* 1971, **21,** 1298.

Zubek, J. B., & Welch, G. Electroencephalographic changes after prolonged sensory and perceptual deprivation. *Science,* 1963, **139,** 1209.

Index